Crack Your Compulsive Eating Code

Charya Hilton

First published 2023 by

Charya Hilton Coaching

www.charyahilton.com

British Library Cataloguing-in-Publication data
A British Library CIP record is available

ISBN 978-1-7393115-0-6
eISBN 978-1-7393115-1-3

Typeset by Tara Evans

Disclaimer
Charya Hilton is not a medical practitioner or certified psychologist. The material in this book is intended for education only. The information given should not be treated as a substitute for medical advice. If you suspect you have an eating disorder or have been diagnosed with an eating disorder, please consult a medical practitioner before engaging in any of the exercises or experiments in this book. Any use of the information in this book is at the reader's discretion and risk. No expressed or implied guarantee of the effects of the use of the recommendations, exercises and experiments can be given or liability taken. Neither the author or the publisher can be held responsible for any loss, claim or damage arising out of the use, or misuse, of the suggestions made, the failure to take medical advice, or for any material on third party websites. Identifying details such as names and locations have been changed to protect privacy.

To my daughters, Tara and Sagara, and my mother, Jean
For your endless love and unconditional support always

CONTENTS

EXPERIMENTS

*Compulsion: a strong feeling of wanting to do something
repeatedly that is difficult to control*
Cambridge English Dictionary

FOREWORD: MY STORY

My personal journey to freedom from my eating and weight issues began when I was in my late twenties, way back in the 1970s. I was depressed, withdrawn, isolated and deeply unhappy. I had been severely anorexic in my late teens which eventually morphed into secretive, compulsive eating, binge eating and bulimia for years after. I was overweight and hated it but I was caught in a never-ending binge/diet cycle, all the while desperately searching for something that would help me overcome my problems and show me how to live a happy, healthy life free from the tyranny of my obsession with food, my weight and my eating problems.

The year I transitioned from anorexia to bulimia I ballooned from five and a half stones (35kg) one Christmas to almost fifteen stones (95kg) the next! I had a massive problem indeed. I saw doctors, psychiatrists, and was prescribed all kinds of diets and diet pills. Nothing worked for long. My weight went down and up so many times I lost count. Now and then I thought I'd cracked it. I would stop binge eating, manage to stick to a diet for a few days and lose a few pounds but then I would blow it and start stuffing myself all over again. It was my dirty little secret and I managed to convince everyone along the way, including my doctors, that I ate like a bird. I only ever binged in secret and even my husband didn't know what I was up to, so I had the added burden of feeling such a liar and a sham. I dreaded being found out.

I was almost at breaking point when a miracle happened. I heard of new women's group for compulsive eaters, and I plucked up the courage to go along. And after that first very nervous evening, I kept on going because I realised I was among wonderful, amazing friends. Those women were like me. They accepted me. They supported me.

I could own up, come clean, come out of my secret eating closet and no-one judged me. I wasn't alone. I wasn't a hopeless case. I wasn't mad, weak or lacking in will power. I wasn't a freak.

As we shared, listened and gently explored our feelings I began to accept I had nothing to be ashamed of and I wasn't guilty of any crime. I had big issues yes, but it wasn't my fault and there was nothing *wrong* with me. I was just trying to deal with stuff I thought I couldn't handle and I had subconsciously developed an eating and piling on weight habit as a coping mechanism.

I began to understand that I could be free from the despair I was enduring if I was prepared to explore what was at the root of my eating behaviour. That inevitably meant feeling feelings – oh my goodness – and on top of that, it meant daring to let go of what wasn't and hadn't been working for years i.e., all the logical ideas I, and every other woman there, held about losing weight. The restrictions, the rules, the security that wasn't really any security at all. The good, the bad and the ugly of dieting.

I decided to go for it. I dedicated myself to discovering all I could about why I couldn't stop eating, why no diet ever worked, why my weight just piled on even though I hated it and the biggest mystery of all – how my eating and weight issues were subconscious attempts to help me avoid what was really at the core of it all by diverting my attention away from my inner world and onto obsessing about my body.

I went into individual therapy digging deep into my life experience past and present looking for clues, patterns and the embedded subconscious codes that were driving me to eat the way I did. I risked expressing my feelings and releasing my emotions rather than numbing them with food or starving to try and deny them. I stopped dieting. I stopped weighing myself. I stopped labelling food as good or bad. I let go of all food restrictions. Over time I gradually reprogrammed myself to trust my body and my natural instincts around food and hunger. I explored how the weight was helping me out – what it was 'saying' for me, how it was creating boundaries I thought I couldn't create for myself, how it was affecting my sexuality, my relationships, my work. And as I gained understanding, said the things I needed to say and made the changes I needed to make consciously, simultaneously the weight, the emotional padding as I came to think of it, gently, naturally, and comfortably let go too. It had no role in my life any more. I stabilised at a size and shape that is just right for my unique body. I've stayed there or thereabouts pretty much all the time since. What I weigh no longer has any meaning for me. Like age, it's just a number. It no longer defines me or affects my mood. I am healthy and happy in my skin. I don't obsess about food or my body any more and food freedom feels so much better than any comfort food tastes!

With my success came a burning desire to help other women crack their personal eating and weight codes too so I studied and trained extensively in therapy, group work, hypnotherapy and coaching and I've worked with hundreds of women individually and in groups since. Helping them to become permanently free from their eating, weight and body struggles and to be the wonderful, powerful, creative, confident, self-assured, self-loving women they are meant to be.

The unique process you will discover in these pages is a synthesis of my personal experience of what really works, my professional expertise and the liberating results that many wonderful courageous women have achieved as my clients, individually and in groups. I am deeply grateful to every woman who has trusted me, and I'm honoured they allowed me to travel their journey alongside them. They taught me so much and without them my dream to reach thousands more women would never have come into being. All names have been changed to protect the honour and privacy of my clients.

May we all be liberated from the tyranny of being at war with food and our bodies and love and accept ourselves from top to bottom forever!

ACKNOWLEDGEMENTS

- To all my clients, individually and in groups, who have trusted me to be their guide as they travelled their personal journey to food freedom. This book would not exist without them. Every person I have had the honour of working with has taught me more than they could ever know and I am deeply grateful
- Susie Orbach without whose amazing, ground-breaking work I would never have started on my own journey to food freedom way back in the late 1970s
- Tara Montane for bringing this book to life with her beautiful design and typesetting skills
- Cheli Grace, the book, business and media strategist helping people become an author of authority, for being my book creation coach, mentor, and motivator
- Ines Padar, aka The Imposter Syndrome Terminator, mindset and business mentor, for encouraging me to overcome my visibility fears and show my authentic self in this book
- Carol Hampshire, brand designer and mentor, for helping me become crystal clear about the heart and soul of my work
- Natalie Ryan Hebert, transformation coach and therapist, for helping me break though my limiting patterns and expand into a greater version of myself
- All the bold, brave, trusting women who gave me permission to share their stories here so others may benefit from them. Their names have been changed to honour their privacy
- The many therapists, trainers, teachers and guides from whom I have learned and whose wisdom has transformed my life – too many to mention here

Thank you

INTRODUCTION

Your eating and weight issues are not the problem,
they are just symptoms of something much deeper...

Crack Your Compulsive Eating Code is designed to help you create a life of food freedom. A life where you feel continuously comfortable around food and permanently happy, confident and secure in your skin. A life you love to wake up to every day!

THIS PROCESS WILL HELP YOU:

* Understand that it's not actually about the food at all!
* Appreciate that your current eating behaviour is not a chronic, incurable condition – it has been an understandable response to various inner and outer pressures which you can learn to respond to differently without resorting to food
* Get to the core of what is causing you to use food for emotional reasons rather than for nourishment
* Allow yourself to feel, and heal, in safety what you have been avoiding by eating and storing weight
* Accept that your weight is subconsciously serving a purpose and until you find out what that is and take on that job consciously it will stick around, or come back after you've lost it, and keep on doing that
* Let go of the self-torture of endless dieting, body shame and self-hatred
* Refresh your body cues around hunger, fullness, and satisfaction
* Learn to trust your body and to eat intuitively as nature intended
* Reprogramme your mind to come to and stabilise at your healthy weight and size forever

The process I am offering you here is the refined, updated, upgraded version of the successful system I used to crack my own compulsive eating code all those years ago. It's the system I've used to help hundreds of women successfully break free from compulsive eating, binge eating, endless unsuccessful dieting and food obsession. It's also helped those women to shed weight naturally, healthily, without dieting and to maintain a healthy weight that is just right for them without effort.

If you are committed and consistent, if you dare to experience feelings you've been avoiding until now and take action based on your discoveries about yourself and your eating behaviour, I assure you, you *will* positively and radically change – for ever! There is no guarantee how quickly that change will happen – you are probably embarking on this adventure because you've had a stressful relationship with food for some time, maybe years, so be patient and loving with yourself.

NO FOOD RULES

Before we get into my top tips for making this process run as smoothly and efficiently as possible, there is one basic principle that underpins it all: there are NO food rules. None. Nada. Zero. Zilch. And, like every woman who has embarked on this journey (including me) you will probably find this the most challenging idea of all. Now I don't expect you to believe that such a seemingly ridiculous notion could ever help you conquer your compulsions and weight issues so all I ask is that you suspend your disbelief for a while and dare to experiment while you proceed through this book.

The No Food Rules of my system are:

No diets. No points. No macros. No numbers.
No sins. No calorie counting. No fasting.
No when you can eat and when you can't. No exercise plans.
No good foods/No bad foods. No good days/No bad days.
No good feelings/No bad feelings.

When clients arrive in my office, they are desperate. They know their weight is the result of their eating behaviour so obviously changing that behaviour – by dieting and restricting food – must be the solution. But even though all of them have been trying for years, it hasn't worked. They often say they feel stupid. Their confidence is at an all-time low. They feel frustrated and angry with themselves because they are generally successful at everything they put their minds to but this one big puzzle has beaten them and it is sapping the joy out of their lives. Some are almost at the point of giving up – but not quite. Some way, somehow, they have heard of my non-diet, food freedom approach and wonder if it might be the answer to their prayers.

They have their doubts of course. My system doesn't make sense. How can letting go of dieting ever help them to lose weight? However, as they are generally at the end of their tether, they have decided to give it a try. Why not? They have nothing to lose – except maybe some weight of course! I set them off on their journey to freedom, that first day we meet, with my top tips for success and here they are for you:

MY TOP TEN TIPS FOR SUCCESS

There may be no food rules but there *is* a system because I want you to be, do, and have what you want in the quickest and most elegant way. I know you. Hanging about isn't your thing, is it? You want results. So, here are my top ten tips for optimum success in this process.

1. **Be kind to yourself.** Be gentle, non-judgemental, speak kindly to yourself. Treat yourself like the goddess you naturally are
2. **Use a dedicated journal.** Buy a new journal or use an empty journal you already have
3. **Go through this book chapter by chapter.** Proceed at a pace that suits you best but proceed. You may want to linger on a particular chapter or experiment or to speed through another but make sure to stick with it as it's intended – don't skip about or step over anything. Just keep going and you WILL transform

4. **Complete all the Code Cracking exercises and experiments.**
    They are designed to consolidate what you learn as you go
    through the chapters

5. **Create a quiet space.** A place to study where you won't be
    disturbed (a room, a corner, on the stairs, in the shed, or even
    in your car if home is a busy whirlwind). If you can dedicate
    a regular time slot of one or two hours each week to your
    study that's great too but you may prefer to split your reading
    time into manageable chunks if that fits your lifestyle better

6. **Listen to your self-hypnosis recording as suggested.** This is
    included in this system. You will find a link and information
    about when and how to listen at relevant times. This
    recording will rewire your mind, overwrite old coding and
    accelerate the positive understanding you gain as you deepen
    and embed your new attitudes to eating, food, your body,
    your weight and your total well-being

7. **Connect with a Code Cracking partner.** It really helps to
    partner up with someone to go through this process with
    you but if that's not possible, find a friend or family member
    willing to listen and support you in a non-judgemental way.
    Having an understanding, accepting, motivating support
    when times get rocky and to celebrate with you when
    positive changes happen works wonders. It may feel scary to
    open up about your problems, especially if you have been
    living a secret eating life, but I found, as many other women
    have, that it can be comforting and liberating to know you
    are not taking this big leap alone. However, if the partnership
    or friend/family member idea is too much to handle right
    now, or ever, it's not essential

8. **Celebrate every step.** The best guarantee of success is positive
    acknowledgement. I know you've been putting yourself
    down, beating yourself up, feeling like you are stuck in this
    eating and weight trap forever, feeling like a failure but you
    can't get this wrong. Ever! We are not going for perfection,
    perfection is unachievable – another finish line always
    appears. We are going for progress over perfection, okay?

9. **Be prepared to feel.** As you crack your coding you may feel things you have denied or suppressed for a while, or even a lifetime. Remember you are always in control and you can stop, take a break and recharge any time you like. A comforting note here: emotions are just energy in motion – E-motion. There are no good feelings and no bad ones. There are just energetic vibrations we prefer and other energetic vibrations we don't like that much

10. **Respect rest.** Transformation takes energy and you may feel more tired than usual at times so if it's possible in your busy life, take rests or short naps if/when you can. I know for women with families, jobs, so much rushing around and organising to do, slotting naps into your schedule might seem an outrageous suggestion but bear it in mind and if you get a moment any time anywhere, take it. Put your head down or rest it back. Shut your eyes and just breathe for a few minutes. It can work wonders.

Relax. You've got this. Just follow the process, fix your eyes on your prize, be consistent and you *will* crack your code and break free from compulsive eating, bingeing, dieting and stressing about your body and your weight forever!

INTRODUCTION KEY POINTS

- It's not about the food. Your eating and weight issues are not the problem, they are just symptoms of something much deeper
- There are no food rules in this process. No diets, no points, no macros, no numbers, no sins, no treats, no calorie counting, no fasting, no when you can eat and when you can't, no exercise plans, no good food/no bad food, no good days/no bad days, no good feeling/no bad feelings
- Emotions are just energy in motion – E-motion. There are energetic vibrations we prefer and other energetic vibrations we don't like that much
- Celebrate every step. You can't get this wrong

CRACK YOUR CODE

1. Buy or prepare your dedicated journal
2. Organise your time and space
3. Set up your code cracking partnership – if you choose to
4. Use the journaling prompts below to get into the habit of journaling:
   a. How do I feel after reading the Introduction?
   b. What doubts do I have? What hopes do I have?

1

IT'S NOT YOUR FAULT!

*Trying to fix compulsive eating with a diet is like trying
to fix a flat tyre with a band-aid.
Add a little pressure and sooner or later it will blow!*

If you are eating compulsively, or binge eating, or eating in secret and have failed over and over to fix your problem with dieting I want you to forgive yourself right now. You've been doing nothing wrong. You're not a failure. You're not a hopeless case with no will power or self-control because none of these problems are fixable with a diet. Each one is a subconscious habit you have encoded into your mind at some point in your life to try and help protect yourself from experiencing feelings you couldn't handle or express. All the diets under the sun could never have worked long term because diets are logical and your eating battles are not logical, they are emotional.

The 'eat less, move more, calories in, calories out results in weight loss' idea seems to make sense if you are unhappy with your eating and your weight. However, emotions override logic every time and when the shit hits the fan, as it always will eventually, the diet flies out the window and there you are once again feeling disappointed and desperate, beating yourself up because you can't stick at it. Maybe you jump back on the diet wagon convinced you must be at fault but rest assured, it won't work for long. When those pesky feelings crop up your emotional protection code will automatically kick in and you'll find yourself alone in the kitchen at midnight, stuffing down biscuits, chocolate, tubs of ice cream, giant sandwiches, or cake wondering 'How did I get here again? What's wrong with me? Why can't I crack this habit?'

HABITS

Habits are subconscious patterns of behaviour that are repeated regularly and through repetition they become encoded into our minds. In other words, we learn them. Every habit is comprised of three components, a cue or trigger, a routine, and a reward.

The cue is what sets the habit off, the routine is what you do while the habit process is operating, and the reward is what this routine has done for you or given you.

Cue > Routine > Reward

In the case of a compulsive eating habit, the process could look like this:

Cue/trigger – a thought, an emotional state you don't like or are anticipating, something someone has said that upsets you, a situation you don't want to deal with, a location you find uncomfortable, etc.

Routine – stuffing choc chip cookies in your mouth, eating cheesecake in your car in secret, eating a huge amount when you're not hungry, eating until you feel sick and over-full

Reward – you feel calmer, emotionally soothed, full, satisfied, maybe sleepy for a while

Now, there is some discussion about how long it takes to embed a habit and the number of repetitions required will vary person to person, but in some cases, if the result is sufficiently rewarding, it may be encoded and become our default mode quite rapidly. In my case, I remember the exact day, time, place, what I was doing, and the feelings I was having when I first triggered my compulsive eating habit into action, and it didn't take many repetitions to get it encoded and working on autopilot. Unfortunately, it kept working far longer than was necessary and any short-term rewards soon turned into long term problems.

These kinds of negative habits always have unintended spin-offs and although for a short while my feelings were soothed each time my compulsion ran its course, it created other unwanted results.

One, the effects didn't last and I had to repeat the process to get a reward that stuck for a while. Two, the result of all that repetition meant it encoded even more strongly each time making it harder to stop. Three, I was gaining weight and that was not what I wanted at all and although I tried to diet to reduce it, eventually that would be too stressful too. And how did I deal with stress? Why with my handy encoded compulsive eating habit of course and so it went around and around until I finally realised what was going on. I set about deleting that code, refreshing my relationship with food, and reprogramming my mind for food freedom and maintaining a happy healthy weight that is just right for my unique body.

SECONDARY GAINS

All habits have secondary gains – one or more additional advantages that come with the basic habit. Subconscious spin-offs that run in-sync with the original coding. With compulsive eating, bingeing and repeated dieting the most common secondary gain is gaining weight! To think that such a problem might have some positive purpose may seem outrageous if you are struggling with it but believe me, it almost always does. For example, the weight and trying to lose it consumes all your attention and diverts you from dealing with your feelings, or it may be acting as a buffer to the outside world, or providing an excuse to not do certain things when you don't have the courage to speak up and say what you do or don't want. It may communicate things about you that you don't dare to say aloud. We will dig into this fascinating aspect of weight and how it may be serving you in detail in a later chapter.

Cracking your compulsive eating code means decoding both bits of the inner game you are running – the emotional rewards of your eating habit and the secondary gains of the weight you have added on in the process. The two operate in harmony and as you release your emotional weight, as you let go and dare to feel, to use your voice, to change what needs to change in your life, you will find that your physical weight will release too and never need to return.

AUTOMATIONS

Our minds are incredible. We can encode habits and beliefs to protect ourselves from emotional harm and distress totally subconsciously. In no time at all they become so efficient they immediately trigger at the slightest whiff of a feeling, a thought, an idea or a situation we find difficult or challenging. Unfortunately, once installed, our codes don't automatically update. If we have subconsciously encoded a compulsion to eat to numb our feelings, our mind will keep repeating that habit even though it may be out of date, way past its usefulness, or harming us into the bargain until we consciously and powerfully choose to do something different.

DIETS DON'T WORK

Right now, millions of people are on a weight loss regime of some kind. Unfortunately, research shows that dieting works for very few of them in the long run: about 95% of dieters will regain any weight they lose, some will gain back even more and many will try the same or a different diet repeatedly and depressingly get nowhere. They buy into the lie that restricting food in some way is the answer, and they think they are at fault, they don't have the will power, there is something wrong with *them*. There isn't!

It is my belief and my personal and professional experience that for a compulsive, emotional and/or binge eater, diets fail over and over because diets are an attempt at an outside fix when solving the problem is essentially an inside job. My inside job, the system I used to crack my compulsive eating code and solve the mystery of how to maintain an easy, comfortable relationship with food and my body – and shed the excess weight and keep it off for good – began to activate the moment I really got it that I had been doing nothing wrong; when I finally accepted I'd just been running a kind of subconscious self-help programme cleverly designed to focus my all my attention on trying to sort the outside whilst the change I was seeking was inside me all the time. I set to work on solving my puzzle from the inside out.

*This process is designed to empower you to do the same
and to create a life you love to wake up to every day!*

CHAPTER 1 KEY POINTS

- You've been doing nothing wrong – diets don't work for most people. Research shows that diets work for very few people in the long run: about 95% of people who go on a diet will regain any weight they lose, and some will gain back even more
- Habits are subconscious patterns of behaviour. A habit is made up of three parts: a cue, a routine (a behaviour), and a reward. Once triggered a habit will run through to the reward automatically
- Every habit has secondary gains – subconscious spin-offs that run in sync with the original code
- Our codes – our embedded habits – don't have automatic updates but we can update, overwrite, and delete them consciously

CRACK YOUR CODE

1. Treat yourself with kindness – do something that makes you feel good. Take a walk, have a bath, read a book, watch something funny on TV, dance, sing in the kitchen – anything that lifts your spirits and fills you with good feelings
2. If you have a code cracking partner, spend up to 15 minutes sharing with them anything you choose about what you have learned so far (feelings, thoughts, ideas, beliefs, disbeliefs, etc.) and then listen to your partner in return. Share as little or as much as makes you feel safe. Please be supportive and non-judgemental. This is a win-win partnership

3.   Try out some of the optional journaling prompts below (as many or as few as you like):

    a.   How do I feel after reading this chapter?

    b.   What doubts do I have? What hopes do I have?

    c.   What is encouraging about this system?

2

WHERE ARE YOU NOW?

*Starting from where you are is the only way
to be sure to get to where you want to be*

To change, to transform, to achieve a goal, to manifest a dream –
whatever way we like to think about it – we need three fundamental
things:

1.   Clarity on where we are now
2.   Clarity on where/who we want to be
3.   A process to get from one to the other

When we set out on any journey, starting from where we are is the
only way to be sure to get to where we want to be. If you turn up
at the wrong airport or station hoping by some magic to get to
your destination regardless, you're going to end up disappointed. So
here and now, you will start your journey to food freedom on the
appropriate platform and the right check in desk – at Stage One.
As your struggles with food and weight are painful and may induce
feelings of guilt and shame, even though you think you are clear
because you tend to focus on your problems most of the time, it may
be that you have avoided being totally honest with yourself. That's
okay. You've been doing nothing wrong but now it's time to own
up and be honest all the while being compassionate with yourself.

STAGE ONE: WHERE ARE YOU NOW?

What is happening for you around food, eating and your weight in
your life? What do you think about yourself? What do you dread
others might be thinking about you? What do you worry about?
How do you use food? What is causing you pain and distress around
food? How is your eating behaviour affecting your life?

Get your journal, get comfortable and maybe have a cup of something if that appeals to you. Answer the following questions, taking as much time as you need. Treat yourself with kindness and as much non-judgement as you can muster and remember, no-one ever needs to know what you write unless you choose to share it so you can be totally honest. Take a breather break or a have stretch any time you want to. The more detailed your answers the better. If any questions don't apply to you and your life, leave them be.

1. What do you think is the most critical thing for you to resolve right now?
2. What do you know you've been doing that isn't working for you?
3. How would you describe your eating habits?
4. What triggers or cues are you currently aware of? What drives you to eat when you're not hungry? For example, when you feel sad/bored/lonely/angry/happy/frustrated/certain situations or circumstances/certain people/when you look in the mirror, etc.
5. What do you think about your eating behaviour?
6. How does your weight and/or eating behaviour affect your self-confidence?
7. What do you think about yourself regarding your weight and eating issues?
8. What do you judge and criticise yourself for?
9. What do you think about your body? What do you judge and criticise?
10. What do you think your weight/body size says about you?
11. What is holding you back from getting the results you want right now?
12. What are your doubts and fears about engaging in this process?
13. Has anyone ever made you feel badly about yourself and your body? If so, what has this made you believe about yourself?
14. What do you wish the young you had been told? If you could go back in time, what would you say to yourself?

When you are done, read back over your answers. How do you feel? However, you feel is fine. Clarity can be mind-blowing I know.

When Emma did this exercise, reading her thoughts and beliefs, seeing them out there on the page was so painful she burst into tears. However, owning up to where she was, what she was doing and how she judged herself all the time brought her to the point where she knew she couldn't go on any longer feeling wretched and hopeless one minute and fooling herself it would all magically work out the next. She was honest and clear about where she was, and she didn't like it. She didn't like it at all. She was ready to start her transformation journey right there and then. Stage One of her transformation was in the bag, or so she thought, but there was more to do yet.

And for you, there is more too. When we have a problem that affects us in so many ways, we tend to focus on all the negative things we think, do and feel. It's as if our struggles consume us and become all of who we are when they are just a fragment. You are so much more than your problem, so much more than your body and there is always an 'also'. You may be in the kitchen at 2am, stuffing food in your mouth as you cry your eyes out in despair but at the same time, you're also a caring, loving woman. You are also kind, thoughtful, brave, have great coping skills, and a genuine desire to be happy and free. You may also be a great mother, sister, aunt, daughter, grandmother, bus driver, friend, artist, athlete, teacher, carer, nurse, dog lover, author, business-woman, singer, dancer, academic, fire fighter, knitter, interior designer, lawyer, shop worker, comedian, cook, charity worker, gardener, musician – the list is endless and none of these qualities and talents disappear because you eat when you're not hungry and maybe carry some weight you don't desire to.

So, for Stage One to be complete I want you to own up to your 'also' qualities too. Get your journal again, settle down and start writing. These journal prompts will help you:

1.   What do you like and love about yourself?
2.   What is important to you?
3.   What values guide you?
4.   What matter to you in the big picture of life?

5. What are your great qualities?
6. What are you good at? What are your talents and skills?
7. What do your family and friends say about you even though you may not believe them?

Again, when you are done, read back over your answers. How do you feel as you recognise and appreciate all the positive values and traits you have? Your 'also' qualities? Some people find this second section of Stage One more challenging than the first as we are not encouraged to acknowledge all that is fine and great about ourselves but with practice it becomes easier.

You see, the transformation you are seeking isn't about changing 'all' of you, a scary prospect indeed. It's more about revealing the natural, authentic you. The you before you gathered all the garbage, beliefs and experiences that have led you to doubt yourself and perhaps even despise your body. As you transform, all your many positive attributes go with you. They are your base, the solid core of you. The 'change' part is just about deleting years of unhelpful coding, letting go of habits that stopped serving you long ago and reprogramming your mind to maintain a healthy relationship with food and your body forever. Your core values, what matters most to you, what you like and love about yourself will remain and become your shining compass as you allow your authentic self to surface and flower. You are already enough; you have always been enough and you will always be enough.

Now relax. Inhale and exhale deeply three times. Roll your shoulders. Shake out your arms and hands. Celebrate and most importantly, congratulate yourself for being so courageous.

Repeat these words, either aloud or inside your head:

> *'I am doing this. I am bold and brave. I am strong.*
> *I am committed. I am amazing because I am cracking*
> *my compulsive eating code, well done me!'*

And notice how you feel about saying this too.

CHAPTER 2 KEY POINTS

- To change, to transform, to achieve a goal, to manifest a dream – whatever way we like to think about it – we need three fundamental things:
  1. Clarity on where we are now
  2. Clarity on where we want to be
  3. A process to get from one to the other
- To crack your personal Compulsive Eating Code, you must start from where you are
- You are so much more than your problem and there is always an 'also'. Own up to your 'also' qualities and acknowledge them
- Celebrate every step. You can't get this wrong

CRACK YOUR CODE

1. Every day, at least once, repeat these words either aloud or inside your head 'I am doing this. I am bold and brave. I am strong. I am committed. I am amazing because I am cracking my compulsive eating code, well done me!'
2. Read your answers to the questions again and allow yourself to feel whatever you feel. Add more information if any appears on your consciousness screen
3. If you have a code cracking partner, share anything you choose to and listen to them in return. Share as little or as much as makes you feel safe. Please be supportive and non-judgemental. This is a win-win partnership
4. Treat yourself with kindness and self-compassion. Take a walk, have a bath, read a book, watch something funny on TV, dance, sing, bake a cake with your kids, cuddle up with a pet, have a coffee chat with a friend on zoom – anything that lifts your spirits and fills you with good feelings

5.   Try out some of the optional journaling prompts below:
     a.   Have I noticed any changes in my eating behaviour so
          far? If so, what?
     b.   What feelings came up when I read my answers to the
          questions?
     c.   What is encouraging about what I've learned in this
          chapter?
6.   When you are ready, move on to the next chapter and create
     your Stage Two

MY WISH IS MY COMMAND

Clarity is the key to being who you want to be

'What do you want? If I could make your dreams come true, what would that look like, how would you feel?' my therapist asked. I felt confused and uneasy. 'I feel stuck and stupid because I can't seem to come up with any answers' I said. 'All the memories of my previous disappointments are getting in the way. I've disappointed myself so many times'.

STAGE TWO: WHO DO YOU WANT TO BE?

Much as you may wish all your dreams could come true, if you've been disappointed many times, being crystal clear on how you want to look and feel, and what you want to be, do and have in your life could be even more challenging than all the coming clean and owning up you have already done. If all your efforts at trying to control your eating have repeatedly ended in defeat, it is natural that you would avoid thinking about specific goals and dreaming of success for fear of feeling all those awful feelings again. To help you breakout of this impasse, some basic information on how the mind works will come in very handy before you go on to create your Stage Two: your 'Dream You'.

YOUR BRILLIANT MIND

Although the mind isn't divided into sections, layers or parts, it can be a helpful model for understanding if we imagine it is but remember, the map is not the territory.

THE CONSCIOUS MIND -10%	THE SUBCONSCIOUS MIND -90%
Can process 40–50 bits of info/second	Can process 11 million bits/second
Short term memory	Long term memory
Thinks and plans	Emotions and feelings
Critical thinking	Incapable of reasoning
Logical thinking	No concept of time
Analyses	Habits, beliefs, patterns, addictions
Tries to control behaviour with willpower	Non-judgemental, flexible
	Creativity, Imagination, Intuition
	Involuntary body functions
	Developmental stages

You can see that most of what we are dealing with in this book – habits, patterns, emotions, feelings – come under the subconscious column, where your programmes and codes are stored. Transformation doesn't happen by just using our conscious mind however much we analyse and try to use our will to get what we want. We need our subconscious mind on side and in alignment with our conscious thinking to create permanent change.

You can work with your mind to your best advantage the more you understand it. Here are the most important things for you to be aware of when it comes to using your mind to achieve your best results.

• Your mind always does what it thinks you want it to do. It doesn't care if what you say is good, bad, true, false, healthy, unhealthy, right or wrong it simply acts on your imagery and words regardless. It follows your commands to the letter

- The mind is hard-wired to keep us safe. To steer us away from pain and towards pleasure. When you're creating your dream, it's important to input pleasurable, alluring, positive, compelling words and imagery to get your mind on your side
- The subconscious mind is the feeling mind. The images we make in our head, the words we say to ourselves and the tone of those words, all affect the way we feel about everything. Feelings drive our actions so always have positive feelings at the core of your dream. Positive images and words create positive habits and actions
- The subconscious mind responds to clear and simple messaging. When you are creating your 'Dream You' make sure you are describing what you *want* to be, do and have – not what you *don't* want. If you can't work out what you want, stating the polar opposite of what you don't want can be a very useful trick to get you out of this dilemma
- The mind is programmed to return to the familiar, and to avoid the unfamiliar. To overcome this programming, fill your vision with familiar feelings of success, pleasure, comfort, safety
- The subconscious mind cannot distinguish between a real and an imagined experience. What you imagine to be happening is actually happening as far as the subconscious mind is concerned
- The subconscious mind has no concept of time. The present is always where it's at for the subconscious mind so use the present tense as you work your magic even though it may seem odd at first
- The mind learns by repetition. You can wire your mind for success by repeating your positive thoughts and imagining your dream over and over. A note here: The same goes for negative thoughts! Repeat them over and over and don't be surprised if you get what you don't want!

WORK YOUR MAGIC: CREATE YOUR STAGE TWO, YOUR 'DREAM YOU'

Now it's time to conjure up your 'Dream You'. Get yourself a cup of something satisfying, have your pen and journal ready. Get comfortable and relax. Take a deep breath and repeat this (either inside you head or out loud) 'I *can* have whatever I want. My wish is my command'. Remember, your subconscious mind follows your commands to the letter so wave your magic wand and tell it exactly what you desire. Spend at least twenty minutes journaling about your wishes and you can have as many as you want. The following prompts can be helpful to stimulate ideas.

- If I could have exactly what I want right now, what would that be?
- How will my life be different when I achieve my dream?
- What will my health be like?
- How will I move? What will I look like? How will I feel in my clothes and without them?
- What will I be doing?
- What will my relationships with my family and friends be like?
- How will I think about food, eating, my body? What will my relationship with food and my body be like?
- And most importantly – *How will I feel?*'

Let your mind run wild and free. Let the genie out of the bottle for up to twenty minutes. When you are finished, come back to this book.

Congratulations! You have your first draft. Read what you have written so far without judgement or the need to get it spot on immediately. Pat yourself on the back. You have taken a big, positive leap that deserves acknowledgement.

CRYSTAL CLARITY: THE KEY TO BEING WHO YOU WANT TO BE

Here are my top tips for crystal clarity and polishing your vision. You can take time out to upgrade your 'Dream You' now or this is included in the Crack Your Code section at the end of this chapter.

1.   Feel it. Check that in your 'Dream You' you are focused on how great you will feel when it materialises. Remember feelings are our greatest drivers. It's the emotion attached to any thought that makes it powerful. If you are stuck for ideas, below are some suggestions you could use. What's your basic 'why' – what feelings are driving you to crack your code? How do you want to feel every day when you wake up?

Joyful	Excited
Sexy	Abundant
Connected	Authentic
Powerful	Positive
Light-hearted	Contented
Confident	Sociable
Intelligent	Compassionate
Fun	Relaxed
Fit	Happy in my skin
Comfortable	Delighted
Relieved	Energetic
Secure	Empowered
Safe	In charge of my life
Fulfilled	Loving
Significant	Passionate
Calm	Peaceful
Worthy	Happy
Enough	Adored
Strong	Boundaried
Self-loving	High self-esteem
Easy around food	Healthy
Relaxed in my clothes	Relaxed without my clothes
Healthy	Honest
Trusting	Open
Free	Authentic

2. Be positive. A positive emotion attached to a positive thought leads to a positive result. Seek out any word, phrase or sentence that isn't useful or positive and delete or change it. Look for confusing information. For example, in her first draft, my client Helen wrote 'I won't bother about what people think of me all the time'. Can you see her sentence was full of sneaky negatives and confusion? We have no idea of what she *does* want to bother about, except that maybe she wants less of bothering about what people think but no specific idea of how much – or if at all. A great start but it's confusing and the subconscious mind can't handle confusing information. I asked Helen to look at it this way: 'Imagine you go on Google and you type in: I know what I don't want so can you find that for me? What do you think Google would come up with?' 'Ah I see', said Helen and after some thought, she upgraded her statement to 'Dressed or undressed I always feel confident, safe and secure in my skin'. No mention of what she didn't want, no ambiguity about time or how much or how often

3. Be present. Write everything in the present tense, as if it is happening right here and now. Change all the *'I wills'* into I *am*, I *have*, I *feel*, I *love*, I'm *excited*, I'm *delighted*, I'm *thrilled* and so on. 'I *will* feel better in my clothes' could simply become 'I feel fabulous in all of my clothes'

4. Focus on what being this version of yourself brings into your life, how it enhances your relationships, your work life, your family life, your health. What it allows you to be, do and have

5. Include your 'also' qualities. You are creating an all-round total image of the person you are choosing to be founded on the authentic you, the core qualities of you that remain and sustain you always, so ensure you include them in your imagery

Now don't be surprised if your 'Dream You' vision makes you feel uncomfortable. This is entirely natural because your disbelief and doubts about how successful you can be are probably hitting the ceiling right now. However, if you understand that this reaction is simply your mind going into overdrive as it tries to pull you back to familiarity mode it will help. Your mind is just doing its job of trying to protect you, trying to steer you away from the pain of feeling another disappointment. When we understand how the mind works it can be so helpful and reassuring to know we don't have to allow our automatic subconscious reactions deter us from achieving our goals and dreams. We can be aware of what is happening and consciously stay focused on communicating to our subconscious mind what we want. We can repeatedly encode what we desire because we know the mind learns by repetition and that repetition will eventually overwrite and crack our old compulsive coding.

RELAX AND DREAM

Rest assured this system will help you clarify, decode, and clear all your doubts and fears as you work through it. All you need to do for the time being is to trust, read your dream often and listen regularly to the self-hypnosis recording that you will find in the resources chapter at the end of this book. This recording is designed to take you on a quantum leap through time and space right into the centre of embodying your dream and the life you long for.

The mind learns by repetition. It also learns most effectively when you are relaxed and enjoying yourself. Listening repeatedly will create the ideal situation for learning as it will help you to relax, it's fun and its full of positive imagery.

Now you have Stage One and Stage Two is coming together. In the next chapters we will work on Stage Three – the system to get from one to the other.

CHAPTER 3 KEY POINTS

- Daring to be crystal clear is the key to arriving where you want to be
- Feelings, emotional states, are the biggest drivers of our actions
- The mind isn't divided into parts or layers, but it is helpful to imagine it is
- The subconscious mind is where transformation happens
- The mind learns by repetition. It also learns most effectively when you are relaxed and enjoying yourself
- The pictures you make in your head and the words you say to yourself shape the way you think about everything
- Celebrate every step. You can't get this wrong

CRACK YOUR CODE

1. Spend time refreshing and upgrading your Dream You. Use my list of the most important things for you to understand and my top tips for polishing your vision. Suspend your disbelief for a while and just go for it. I want you to aim for the most incredible results and wonderful, exciting 'Dream You' you can imagine. Keep upgrading as often as you like as you learn more and progress through this system
2. Read your 'Dream You' at least once every single day and imagine being her now
3. Listen to your self-hypnosis recording: The Quantum Jump once each day or evening or just before sleeping until you have listened to it at least 21 times. Listen in a quiet place where you won't be disturbed. Turn off or silence all technology, phones, tablets etc. Do *not* listen while driving or operating any kind of machinery. If you fall asleep that's fine. You mind will accept the suggestions as your subconscious mind never sleeps. You will find a link to download this recording in the resources section at the end of this book

4. If you have a code cracking partner, share anything you choose and listen to them in return. Share as little or as much as makes you feel safe. Please be supportive and non-judgemental
5. Treat yourself with kindness and compassion
6. Try out some of the optional journaling prompts below – as many or as few as you like:
    a. How did I feel as I created my dream?
    b. What would I have to believe about myself to be that dream me?
    c. What was difficult? What doubts came up, what challenged me?
    d. What is encouraging about what I've learned in this chapter?
7. When you are ready, move on to the next chapter and start working the system

Just for fun … If you think you can't make pictures in your mind, here are some optional, easy games that will boost your confidence. Reading through each game first and then try it.

a. My Front Door

Sit comfortably and close your eyes. Take a breath or two and begin to imagine the front door of your house or the door to your flat (or the entrance you usually use to enter your home). Allow the image to gradually become clearer, notice the shape, the colour(s), and any features that tell you it's your door. Is there a knocker, a bell, a letterbox? Where is the lock or the handle you use to open it? What does it look like?

Now keeping your eyes closed, imagine you are about to go in. Reach out and put your imaginary key in the imaginary lock or reach for the imaginary door handle. See your door and see or sense your hand turning the key or the handle. Open the door and go inside. Take a good look around and see what you see. Then slowly open your eyes.

What happened? Did you get a clear picture or even a glimmer? I bet you saw something otherwise how would you know where to go home to? Your vision may have been a bit fuzzy or out of focus, but you can improve with practice. The next game will help.

b. An Object in Mind

Choose either your pen or your journal for this game. Whichever one you choose, pick it up and spend a few moments examining it in detail. Place it in front of you. Look at it from a distance and then close-up. See it from different angles, from above and below. Notice the shape, colour(s), all its features.

When you think you have every detail, close your eyes and imagine it, picture it. See its shape, colour and all the other details you noticed. When you have had a good look with your 'inner eyes', open your eyes. Again, what happened?

If your results in these games were not as clear as you would like, relax. Not everyone finds it easy at first to see images in detail. Practice them again and see what effect that has or create some games of your own.

4

IT'S NOT ABOUT THE FOOD

*Your issues with food have nothing to do with food
– it's what you are using food for that's the issue*

On my journey to food freedom, I discovered many interlinked, subconscious factors were playing a part in preventing me being the woman I wanted to be. All were doing their bit to try and help me solve situations and conflicts I thought I couldn't handle, to submerge feelings I was frightened to feel, to provide a buffer and boundaries, to protect me in some way. I recognised I had been using food to try and solve multiple problems it is not designed to do. Food cannot solve problems – but eating can sure create plenty!

Compulsive eating is a complex, multi-layered issue. To get from Stage One to Stage Two, your Dream You, it's not enough to simply know where we are and have a wonderful vision about where and who we want to be. If that was all it took, most of us would have solved our problems long ago. No, we need a practical, tried and tested system to get from one to the other. This and the following chapters provide you with the system I used to crack my compulsive eating code and it's the system I have used to successfully support many women over many years to refresh their relationship with food and reprogramme their minds to come to and maintain their healthy, happy weight forever.

The experiments in this chapter are the foundation upon which everything else will build so please honour yourself and your commitment by fully engaging in each one as I suggest. Become a detective looking for the clues, patterns, connections, thoughts and feelings which will reveal your personal food and eating codes. Until you're crystal clear about what you've been doing and what's not been working, you will be stuck in the dark and at the power of your subconscious mind. Dig deep, dare to be honest, expose your heart and soul and the gains will be phenomenal because with understanding comes power – the power to transform and to heal. And, as before, no-one need ever know what you discover unless you choose to share it so you can let it all out at last. In later chapters you will experiment with how to safely express your feelings, build new habits, trust in your natural body cues and how to piece it all together and reprogramme your mind to maintain a healthy weight forever. For now, let's start with the basics.

Remember, a habit plays out like this:

> **Cue/trigger** – a thought, an emotional state you don't like or are anticipating, something someone has said that upsets you, a situation you don't want to deal with, a location you find uncomfortable etc.
>
> **Routine/behaviour** – stuffing choc chip cookies in your mouth, eating cheese rolls in your car in secret, eating a lot when you're not hungry, eating until you feel sick and over-full, etc.
>
> **Reward** – you feel calmer, emotionally soothed, full, satisfied, maybe sleepy for a while.

Even though it may be painful to focus on what you're currently doing in your food and eating life, it is the only way to guarantee success in becoming your Dream You. The temptation to deny and ignore reality is great I know, you are an expert at that already, but delay, procrastination and repeating what you've been doing for years isn't working is it so let's get cracking.

Your first experiment *The Seven Day Eating Log* follows. Please remember that the purpose of your detective work is to gain clarity and understanding *without* judgement, guilt, or shame. You haven't committed any crimes and you've been doing nothing wrong okay? You are not guilty, and you have nothing to be ashamed of. You have simply been trying to deal with situations, relationships, and emotions you believe you can't handle so be kind and gentle with yourself all the way through and especially, be patient. It takes time and repeated practice to change habits and it is natural to falter and stumble sometimes.

EXPERIMENT ONE: THE SEVEN DAY EATING LOG

Right now, I'm not suggesting you try to change anything. No demand to ditch your diet or let go of all your food rules yet. In this experiment you are simply looking for cues and clues about what you are currently doing and thinking. Your goal is to gain understanding because understanding is power. Your task is to log the times, cues/triggers, behaviour, and results for everything you eat and drink for seven days. Every single meal, snack, nibble, drop and mouthful that passes your lips however small and insignificant it may seem. The column headings on the table overleaf give you all the information you need to fill in your log. You will need seven copies, one for each day. You can make copies in your journal or download copies via the link in the Resources section at the end of this book.

Note: this is called The Seven Day Eating Log not the calorie counting, macro numbers, sins, treats, good/bad foods log or what do I weigh or how fat/thin am I log. You will see that none of these factors are included because it's not about the food it's about your thoughts, your feelings and your habits. Now I understand that it may be tempting to do all that counting and measuring because that's diet culture programming and it can be difficult to drop but avoid it as much as you can. And if it happens, it happens. Be aware of it and recognise that it is just another conditioned code that's all. Remember. As you fill in your columns aim for no guilt, no shame, just curiosity. However, if those emotions arise just note when and where they occur. Record any discoveries in your journal as you go through the days. What patterns can you see? Which feelings, situations, interactions, people, thoughts, places tend to trigger you the most? Are there certain times of day or evening or night that are noticeably challenging? Do you reach for, or feel drawn to, particular foods or food groups at those times? What feelings result from different eating experiences?

Date:

Time	What was I thinking? Was I hungry? What was going on?	How was I feeling before eating?	Where did I eat?

What and how I ate	Did the food satisfy me or not?	Feelings after eating

After her seven days of logging Candice said,

'I've had a great week. I've used the log religiously which has already stopped me from picking while I'm cooking, I didn't realise how much I did that! It's also made me aware of when I'm snacking and that I'm often eating when I'm not hungry. I notice when I get bored or annoyed about something or someone or I feel lonely, I end up at the fridge and I usually go for something sweet and creamy. I also realise that I'm angry with myself for not standing up for myself more. I think I'm a bit of a push over. A real people pleaser'.

THE POWER OF OUR THOUGHTS

Our thoughts create our feelings, our feelings drive our actions, our actions create our habits and our habits create our results. It all begins with our thinking and if we want to change what we are doing and getting, it pays to start at the beginning, by becoming aware of our thoughts. The Eating Log reminds you to focus on your thinking first because those thoughts are crucial to what does or doesn't happen next. After a week or so of logging, often you can see certain thoughts arise frequently and that they are cues that set particular habits running over and over again. I wonder what thoughts and consequent actions you will discover as you complete your seven-day log!

WHAT WAS I THINKING?

We say, 'What was I thinking?' so often don't we? And usually in a judgemental way when something goes wrong, or we do something we didn't want to or maybe feel a bit silly or stupid about. We say these words without really listening to ourselves or realising what a great question it is. I want you to get into the habit of asking yourself 'What am I thinking?' or 'What was I thinking?' regularly, with curiosity, and *non-judgementally* from now on. You see we can choose our thoughts and when we do that, we can have agency over our actions. We don't have to keep running on automatic pilot always ending up right back where we started countless times. We can choose new thoughts that help us get to where we really want to be.

The following experiement is designed to create a 'stop and notice your thoughts' habit.

EXPERIMENT TWO: STOP! WHAT AM I THINKING?

So, let's imagine you find yourself mindlessly ending up at the fridge when you aren't hungry, or standing in the kitchen at night shovelling ice cream down your throat not really knowing how you got there, or driving your car to the nearest service station to get a big bar of chocolate or three to eat in secret in the dark. In those moments when you realise you're doing the same old, same old thing over again, I want you to remember to do this simple experiment. It only takes a minute or two of your time, but it is very powerful.

This is how it goes:

1. **Stop!** The moment you realise you are on the brink of repeating an old habit, simply stop. Stop what you are doing. Take a breath or two and be still (of course, if you're driving, pull over somewhere safe first!). Then in that still moment, ask yourself:

2. **What am I thinking?'** What words am I saying to myself? What images are coming to my mind? What am I telling myself about who I am and what I can do, cope with, handle etc.? (You may find it useful to have a recording app on your phone for any 'live' experiments in this book so you can record your thoughts and feelings instantly but it's not essential). Next, ask yourself:

3. **What am I feeling?** Am I feeling upset, sad, angry, lonely, bored, excited, hopeless, overwhelmed, jealous, frustrated? Next, ask yourself:

4. **What physical sensations am I experiencing?** 'What am I feeling in my body?' e.g., tightness, pain, tiredness, aches, breathless, heart racing, etc. Next do nothing except:

5. **Honour your thoughts and feelings** by giving yourself time to breathe and register and acknowledge your experiences. Next take a few slow, deep breaths and:

6.   **Imagine the woman you are dreaming of being,** focus your mind on that image you have of yourself. Imagine she is right there in front of you and now ask yourself:

7.   **What would she do?** What would she do when she finds herself in this situation? Allow those thoughts and ideas to come up on your consciousness screen and whatever emerges, now you do that! **Take action!**

Note: If you find it difficult to do what 'she' would do or to work that out, first congratulate yourself for doing this experiment. You are brave and bold and deserve applause, so give yourself a break. Then move. Move away from where you are to another place in the room, or to a different room, or drive somewhere else, or go for a walk. Move your body*. Do something, go somewhere different and wait patiently until you have some inkling of what she would do. And, when you get that inkling, do your best to do that. You know that thing when you lose your car keys and you give up searching then, lo and behold, you suddenly remember where you left them? Well like that. Allow the answer to emerge by itself, no pressure no stress.

   * If mobility is difficult for you, stretch or twist in some way, or reach
     your arms out or move your feet or shake your hands vigorously.
     Anything that gets the blood moving.

I often suggest to my clients that they practice 'Stop! What am I thinking?' regularly, when they are not in a stress eating situation. That way they become so familiar with the procedure that when the shit hits the fan it comes easily to mind and they know exactly what to do. Also, it can be fascinating to catch our thoughts and see what effect they may be having on our experience day to day.

What comes out of your mouth is as important as what goes into it when it comes to cracking your compulsive eating code. The next experiment will focus your attention on how you speak about youself.

EXPERIMENT THREE: WHAT AM I SAYING?

How do you speak about yourself every day? How would you describe yourself to someone else? Do you speak harshly to yourself? Do you criticise yourself? Would you speak to a friend, a relative, your child, a co-worker in the same ways?

I want you to remember always that the little girl we once were still lives deep inside all of us. Every time you criticise or speak harshly to yourself, she hears it and she feels it. So, from this moment on I want you to become aware of your internal dialogue and the words that come out of your mouth. Make a declaration to yourself now that you will monitor your language and dare to speak lovingly to yourself however hard that might be. You know, you cannot hate yourself slim. You've tried that and it hasn't been working for you, has it? So, it's time to experiment with another approach and crack your negative self-description code.

YOUR DECLARATION: I declare that I will pay attention to how I speak to myself internally and what comes out of my mouth as I describe myself to myself, and to others. I will crack my code of negative talk and dare to speak lovingly to myself and about myself. As the mind learns by repetition, keep repeating your declaration and acting upon it until you overwrite your old coding and a new positive speaking code becomes hardwired and your natural default.

After making her declaration, Susan told me she was shocked to realise how often she criticised herself. She noticed that whenever she looked at herself in the mirror, she was mentally saying 'I hate my fat stomach. My arms are flabby and disgusting. My double chin is awful, it makes me look so old. My clothes look terrible on me'. She took a bold leap and decided to start saying something different. As saying positive words about her body was a stretch at first, instead of focusing on how she looked, she started by focussing on who she was. She told me that when she caught herself about to say something negative, she stopped and said, 'I'm a beautiful person. I am I'm a great friend. I'm a wonderful mum. I'm great at my job'. Another time she said, 'I may want to shed some weight but this body has been carrying me around for years and however much I've spoken harshly to it or not treated it well, it's still here, and it's still working for me'. Gradually over time, it became easier to slip in some positive descriptions of her body too. She said, 'I heard your voice in my head saying it's not about going for perfection. It's about going for progress. And I am progressing every day. Every single time I speak kindly to myself I know I'm rewiring my mind; I'm cracking my code step by step'

EAT PEOPLE

A therapist once gave me another way out of a compulsive eating situation that didn't involve any thought investigation, logging or imagining what my dream me would do. She said, 'When you find yourself in that desperate moment of feeling compelled to eat even though you know you aren't hungry and all you're doing is trying to avoid an emotion, an uncomfortable situation, or your avoiding saying or doing something you want to but feel you just can't, don't eat *food*. Eat *people*'. Of course, she didn't mean become a cannibal. What she meant was communicate with somebody, speak to somebody, connect with somebody because very often what we're missing in these moments is connection.

Now I know from my own experience that the last thing we feel like doing at these times is to talk to somebody. I felt ashamed and guilty enough already and the idea of telling someone else what I was doing, or about to do, and maybe have them judge me was horrifying, so I discounted my therapist's advice as a bit stupid. She obviously hadn't been in my situation or she would know how impossible it was. Then one day I realised I didn't have to tell anyone *what* I was doing or about to do. My wise therapist didn't mean that. All she meant was that I just needed to connect.

I could call my bestie and chat about what I had been binge watching on Netflix. Or call a relative and ask them how they were doing. Or meet a friend in a café and put the world to rights. Or sit down on the ground with a homeless person and chat about the weather. It didn't matter who or where or what, and I never need talk about my food and eating problems if I didn't want to. I just needed to get out of the situation I was in, take the focus off myself and the emotional steam out of what I was doing or about to do. Eventually, I plucked up the courage. I ate people and, you know what? It worked. Not always. Sometimes I just didn't have the nerve or the energy to put down the food and pick up the phone but when I did, I felt so much better.

Eating people wasn't a magic bullet. It didn't solve all my problems overnight, but in those moments or sometimes hours of connection, I forgot about myself for a while. I often returned home or came off a call feeling more in charge of my life and almost always feeling more positive and hopeful. Through my therapist I met another woman on the food freedom journey too and we became calling partners. That was life-changing as she and I shared similar problems and challenges. We were ready to listen, to support and to motivate each other as we practiced our experiments. She helped me step away from the fridge countless times and it was liberating to feel I could be honest without being judged. We gained courage and power from each other, and I am eternally grateful that she was and still is in my life.

The following experiment is about how to eat people rather than food.

EXPERIMENT FOUR: EAT PEOPLE

If you find yourself feeling compelled to eat when you know you are not hungry, your emotions are running high and the idea of watching your thoughts or noticing what you are saying or filling in your Eating Log is all too much to handle, be bold. Don't eat food. Eat people. Reach out. Connect with somebody. Connect with your code cracking partner if you have one. Speak to somebody in your house or if there's nobody there or you don't want to, phone a friend or go out and meet someone for coffee. Anything that gets you connected with another person or people will do. Then just chat. Chat about anything. Calm down. Let the steam out and relax. (I have gone out and chatted to the checkout person in my supermarket or to someone at the bus stop in the past when I couldn't find anyone else willing or able to chat with me).

When the conversation or the meet-up is over, notice if you come off the call or return home feeling calmer and the burning desire to eat has passed – even briefly. Even if it hasn't, you have given yourself space. You didn't react automatically. You tried something different and you began to crack the code that triggers you to eat when you're feeling overwhelmed or emotional. Remember whatever happens, congratulate yourself every time for being bold and brave and committed to solving your problems. Speak kindly to yourself.

CHAPTER 4 KEY POINTS

- Your issues with food have nothing to do with food. It's what you're using for food for that's the issue
- The only way to get to where you want to be, is to understand and accept what's going on in your current food and eating life
- The purpose of your detective work is simply to gain clarity and understanding *without* judgement, guilt or shame
- The Eating Log is not about the food, it's about your thoughts, feelings and eating habits
- Thoughts create our feelings, our feelings drive our actions, our actions create our results. Every habit of action is a habit of thought first
- What comes out of your mouth is as important as what goes into it
- Eat people, not food when you are in a food stress situation
- Celebrate every step. You can't get this wrong

CRACK YOUR CODE

1. Complete seven days – at least – of Experiment One: The Seven Day Eating Log and journal about your discoveries
2. Practice Experiment Two: Stop! What Am I Thinking?
3. Practice Experiment Three: What Am I Saying? and repeat your declaration: I declare that I will pay attention to how I speak to myself internally and what comes out of my mouth as I describe myself to myself, and to others. I will crack my code of negative talk and dare to speak lovingly to myself and about myself
4. Practice Experiment Four: Eat People when you feel an episode of food stress coming on or you are on the brink of one

5. If you have a code cracking partner, spend time sharing anything you choose to and listen to them in return. Share as little or as much as makes you feel safe. Please be supportive and non-judgemental
6. Listen to your self-hypnosis recording: The Quantum Jump once each day or evening or just before sleeping (the choice is yours), until you have listened to it at least 21 times. If you fall asleep that's fine
7. Treat yourself with kindness and compassion
8. When you are ready, move on to the next chapter and start cracking your emotional codes

FEELINGS

Food isn't magic – it cannot make feelings disappear

You are an intelligent woman. You know food isn't magic yet, somehow, you've bought into the illusion that it is and you've given food a power it doesn't have. I bought into the illusion too. I discovered I could instantly bury any old feeling I didn't like with a few cakes and a couple of bars of chocolate. And if the feeling seemed to be creeping back up, piling in more chocolate, ice cream, crisps, cake, biscuits, cheese sandwiches and anything else I could lay my hands on would do the trick. Very quickly I developed a habit. Food became my drug of choice, helping me to feel comfortably numb. I didn't know back then that my feelings were simply mental and physical messengers trying to make me aware of something that needed attention.

I believed in food magic because for a while it seemed to be helping me out but pretty quickly I began developing another problem that the magic couldn't fix; my expanding body. Now I had a major dilemma. I felt compelled to eat because I wanted to numb my feelings, but that habit was causing another issue, my weight, which then became the focus of all my despair.

I struggled to fix my weight with diet after diet but should an inkling of a discomforting feeling arise, boom! The diet went out the window in an instant. My eating compulsion kicked in and ruined my every attempt to lose weight. I would find myself back at the fridge or searching in the cupboards, eating in secret, crying, feeling hopeless and a failure. However much I ate, the magic no longer worked. I felt dreadful most of the time, ensnared in a never-ending cycle of compulsive eating and endless dieting.

Thankfully, I discovered a way out of the trap. No false magic, no tricks, no illusions would be involved but I would have to be prepared to feel, to express my feelings and deal with the consequences. I had to finally accept that what I had been doing wasn't working – and would never work because my weight and my eating issues were symptoms of something deeper. My therapist gave me the Eating Log and various other experiments to complete. Just like you that was how I began. Next, I learned how to safely express and release those feelings rather than automatically and subconsciously shifting into my default code of 'try to bury or numb them with food'. Later in this chapter you will learn how to express your feelings healthily and safely too, but first let's understand how you've been trying to use food magic because understanding is power.

FOOD MAGIC – HOW HAVE YOU BEEN USING IT?

With curiosity, and showing compassion and kindness to yourself, from your experiments in the previous chapter what have you discovered so far? What feelings and thoughts have you been trying to bury, numb or avoid with your food tricks? Here are some responses other women have shared with me.

Anger	Fear	Shame	Guilt	Sadness
Resentment	Boredom	Loss	Secrecy	Jealousy
Envy	Despair	Stuck	Excitement	Frustration
Joy	Rage	Loneliness	Grief	Pain

Feeling excited	Stopping myself doing something
Fear of success	Fear of disappointing someone
Feeling I'm 'too much'	Coping with my unhappy relationship
Hopelessness	Feeling not good enough
Feeling different	Fear jealousy from others
Fearing rejection	Scared to speak my mind
Fear of being alone	Fear of abandonment
Work stress	Dumbing down my creativity
Fear of failure	Money worries

I have to go along with what other people want

Now, all those feelings you've been trying to magic away with food haven't disappeared. They have just gone somewhere else. If we prevent a feeling from surfacing, it will appear in some other way. For example, suppressed anger is one of the most common feelings recognised by women I work with after completing their Eating Log. All that suppressed anger doesn't go anywhere but in because it can't come out. You may try to eat it away – but you end up getting angry with yourself as you pile on the pounds as a kind of internal, subconscious pay-back for not daring to say what you need to say or doing what you need to do. That anger you hope you're burying or denying is just being stored as emotional weight around your body until you dare to give it the respect it deserves.

Like any feeling, anger is only energy moving but many of us have been taught there is an embargo on expressing anger or any other so-called negative emotion. We are given the impression, or perhaps even told explicitly, that such feelings are dangerous, destructive, overwhelming, engulfing, unmanageable, even unladylike forces, but they are only so if they are forbidden or not permitted. And it's not only the negative ones either. 'Don't get too excited, it will all end in tears' was a saying frequently bandied about by my mother when I was a child. It confused me because no-one ever explained what 'too excited' meant or how I could gauge it. And tears, obviously that was a bad thing to happen although I didn't understand why as apparently it was fine for my mother to blub profusely over a schmaltzy film on TV. It took me years to let myself get excited, really, truly, full-on excited, and you know what? It never did end in tears but even if it had, it would have been worth it. You will have your own feeling embargoes and it can be enlightening to take a trip down memory lane and see what sayings and utterings whizzed around the rooms of your childhood and what effect they may have had on your life. Without blame or judgement of course, just with curiosity for the purpose of understanding.

WHAT DID YOU LEARN FROM YOUR EATING LOG?

Feelings are there to be experienced. To be felt. They tell us we are alive in all our many ways and trying to hide or stifle them negates that aliveness and we suffer in some way as a result. Get your journal, your pen, your Eating Log pages, a cup of something satisfying and spend some quality time with yourself reviewing you Log and answering the following prompts. As always, be curious, not judgemental.

a. What appear to be the most common reasons or triggers for me to binge or eat compulsively or feel driven to eat?
b. What predominant thoughts and feelings are cropping up in my Eating Log?
c. What emotions or feelings do I seem to find the most difficult to feel and/or express?
d. Where am I most likely to be when I find myself eating compulsively?
e. When am I most likely to eat compulsively?
f. When do I seem to find it most challenging to express myself?
g. Who or what seems to trigger me into eating compulsively?
h. Who comes to mind that I would like to speak to about anything I have noticed so far?
i. How do I feel about speaking to that person?

Your next experiment will help you gain more clarity on the cues compelling you to eat rather than feel.

EXPERIMENT FIVE: WHAT WOULD HAPPEN IF?

Read through this experiment before you begin and when you are familiar with the process, close your eyes and sink into it. Or, even better, record it onto a device. Please make sure you will not be disturbed while you are relaxing. You may want to refer to your Eating Log before fully engaging in the experiment.

1. Settle down in a comfortable chair or on a bed with your hands and feet uncrossed. Take some deep breaths, relax, and close your eyes

2. Now, allow your mind to drift back slowly and gently to a challenging time in the last seven days when you remember feeling compelled to eat even though you knew you weren't hungry

3. Drift back to that scene .. and just be there now. Be right inside it, as if it is vividly happening this moment

4. In this scene, is it daytime or night-time? Are you inside or outside? Are you alone or is someone else with you?

5. Where are you? What can you see and hear?

6. Now focus on what is happening **just before you start to eat** – what's going on? What are you saying/not saying, doing/not doing? If there are other people in this scene, what are they saying/not saying, doing/not doing? How are you feeling? What are you thinking?

7. Is this a familiar scenario/feeling/sensation? Or is it a one-off?

8. Is this a time/place/situation/difficulty that tends to make you resort to food?

9. Focus all your attention on your emotional state **just before you start to eat.** Can you give this emotional state a name?

10. Let whatever you are feeling come to the surface now and in this situation, is there something you want to say or do but feel you can't, shouldn't, or don't dare to?

11. Now imagine that instead of eating, you just let yourself feel what you were feeling just before you started eating

12. What do you fear would happen if you let yourself express that feeling or say what you want to say?

13. When you are ready, come back to now

For the nineteen years of their marriage, Janet always went along with what her husband Tim wanted regarding evening mealtimes even though she didn't want to. Tim was a great cook and cooked most nights and Janet loved that he cooked so often. He was a caring husband and father and they shared parenting equally. She had nothing to complain about she told me, and she felt guilty raising the subject of their evening meals because she felt so lucky compared to most of her friends. However, Tim cooked the kind of food she didn't really like. She had an Italian background and preferred lots of fresh vegetables, pasta and lighter foods served up in dishes so you can choose what you want and how much. Tim tended to cook meat heavy, stodgy food and always served it up on the plate, never giving her the opportunity to decide what and how much she wanted. To please him, she mostly ate everything he gave her even if she felt stuffed.

Janet knew this situation wasn't helping her weight issues but after completing her Eating Log, she became even clearer because she noticed that even though she was full after the heavy evening meals, she often ended up snacking at night trying to swallow down the anger she felt at herself for not daring to speak up. She realised that her weight problems were not so much about the evening meals but more about not feeling she could ask for what she wanted.

Janet found the idea of talking to Tim challenging because she didn't want to upset him. After all she was lucky compared to most

CONFLICTING THOUGHTS

Conflicting thoughts get in the way of our progress because they confuse our mind. The mind cannot process conflicting ideas, they cancel each other out and we end up wondering why we feel stuck. Some examples of conflicting thoughts in the compulsive eating arena might look like:

'I don't want to be fat – but I want to belong in my family, and they are all fat so I have to be fat because if I'm not fat I'll feel different and I won't belong'

of her friends. If she told him what had been going on for all their married life, she was worried he would take anything she said the wrong way. However, with her new understanding, she realised she'd been compromising herself for far too long and it was time to either take a risk or to keep eating in the kitchen at night and keep increasing her weight. She bided her time until one evening, when they were comfortable and cosy together, she plucked up her courage and gently and carefully explained what had been going on for her. She felt nervous but she was pleasantly surprised because all Tim said was 'Why have you never told me that? I had no idea because you never said anything! Of course, it's fine. I'll cook what I like sometimes and what you like at other times. That's easy to work out and you know me. I'll eat anything! And if you don't want me to serve up the food, I never need to do that again. You can always choose as much as you want'. And that's just what happened from then on.

Janet realised she had been living in fear of a fantasy and that gave her the courage to go on to challenge other habits, patterns and beliefs. Not everything was as easy as the evening meals saga but she knew each time she dared to do, say, or feel what she needed to, her need for food magic waned and eventually disappeared altogether. She created new codes to cancel out the old and reprogrammed herself to eat in a way that gently took her to her natural, healthy weight and she has remained there ever since.

'I want to be slim but I'm not willing to say/do/feel what I know I need to say/do/feel to achieve that'

'I want to be fit and healthy but I'm just not worth the effort because I feel so bad about myself'

'I want to be slimmer but that means I will be more attractive and I don't know how to fend off the advances of men so staying overweight means I'll avoid that problem'

Daphne said,

'I want to lose weight and I try endlessly, but I realised that I'm continuously giving my mind confusing information. You see, every single Saturday all the female members of my family are expected to gather in my mother's house for tea, and I hate it. They always talk about their weight. Everyone is overweight, always on some diet or another. Like me, no-one ever succeeds in their dieting – but they go on and on about how fat they are, and how hopeless it all is really because obviously it's genetic. They all have a weight problem they can't fix however hard they try, so it must be, they say. From my Eating Log I realised three things about these gatherings. One: I really don't want to go but I'm scared of my mother's reaction. Two: I notice I always eat a lot before I go – to calm myself down, I think. Three: I think staying overweight makes me feel like I belong. I'm not different, I'm one of the family even though I don't want to be there, I don't want to talk about dieting, and I don't want to be overweight'.

Isn't this interesting! Can you see all the conflicting threads of thoughts, feelings and actions that add up to Daphne feeling stuck and confused? I wager you can guess exactly what Daphne could do to ease her situation and make the changes she says she want to make, but can you also understand the challenges she faces in doing so? Have you noticed any conflicting thoughts in your personal research?

It can be very helpful to use your inner child as a guide and focus for your best intentions and well-being. Yes, she is always present. You may have forgotten about her, but she hasn't gone anywhere except deep inside. You carry her with you always. The next experiment is very simple.

EXPERIMENT SIX: LOVING YOUR MINI-YOU

1. Close your eyes and imagine yourself as being about six or seven, or even younger if you prefer
2. Imagine that little mini-you is right there in front of you and now imagine you can gently pick her up and put her on your lap
3. Now imagine giving her a hug and smelling her hair and feeling the warmth and the weight of her little body. Isn't she lovely and delightful?
4. Become familiar with her and enjoy her sitting there on your lap for a while
5. Say some kind and loving words to her inside your head. Imagine you are the most loving parent she could ever have and tell her how bright, funny, gorgeous, lovely, delightful she is
6. Now I want you to vow that from now on it will be your number one job to take care of your little mini-you in the very best way you can
7. Sense her on your lap and make a promise to her that you will check in with her needs whenever you feel you are about to eat compulsively or mindlessly because you can't face, or don't dare to express your feelings
8. Make a promise to her that in those moments of choice, you will stop and ask yourself, as the adult in this partnership, what good will this do my dear, sweet little mini-me? Will it care for her? Will it help her to be happy, healthy and well? Will it let her know that her feelings are messengers I am paying attention to in healthy ways?
9. When you have your answer, you make the choice in that moment that serves your little mini-me best

If you keep your promise, guess what? Every time you check in and do just that, you will be deleting years of unhelpful and maybe harmful coding and installing new codes of self-love and self-care by default.

FEEL IT

We can harbour difficult feelings like grief, sadness, anger, fear, jealousy for years and never let ourselves feel or express them. However, as we know, these feelings don't magically go anywhere because we deny or bury them. They just bubble away under the surface. Sometimes speaking up or doing something isn't the solution – we just need to give ourselves the space to experience them and nothing more. To allow the feeling to surface, to pass through us, and to let it go. With practice, we can become familiar with our feelings and accept that they won't destroy, overwhelm, or consume us.

Experiment Seven allows you to feel in a gentle, caring way.

EXPERIMENT SEVEN: SPACE TO FEEL WHAT YOU FEEL
Read through the experiment first.

1. Sit comfortably in a quiet place by yourself and maybe have some tissues handy
2. Close your eyes and let your mind drift back to the last time you didn't express a feeling
3. Go back to that moment, that time, that experience, that place and just relive it in your mind
4. Give the feeling time and space to come up or show up or bubble up
5. Can you give the feeling a name? Can you speak that name out loud?
6. Say I feel .... (I feel alone, I feel angry, I feel sad, I feel jealous etc., you fill in the gaps with your words)
7. Now just sit with what you feel. Allow it to just be there for as long as you can
8. Saying the name of the feeling aloud or even inside your head honours it and helps it to pass through you and release more easily
9. Your task is to let your feeling arise, to name it, to allow it to flow through you and then to release it and let it go. If you need to come back to any event and repeat this experiment again, because you feel there is more to release, that's fine
10. Set aside some time each week to practice this experiment and show gratitude to your feelings as they are a sign of your aliveness

Sometimes allowing a feeling to flow through you needs some encouragement or the feeling just feels stuck and needs definite action. The next experiment will help you get your feelings moving.

EXPERIMENT EIGHT: LET IT RISE AND LET IT OUT

This experiment is a safe way to release strong emotions like anger and your little mini-you will love it! You can try all or some of the versions. Whatever version you choose, you can be by yourself or have someone supporting you. It's up to you. Be somewhere where you feel safe emotionally and physically, where there is some space and no objects that might get in your way. A bedroom can be a good place or outside in the fresh air is great too. Read through the experiment before trying it and maybe have some tissues handy. You can choose one or any number of the options below.

1.   Begin by remembering a time when you held in a strong feeling. Allow that time to come vividly to mind. When you are ready, choose any one of the options below:

   a.   Start stamping your feet on the ground and let your stamping grow stronger as you say aloud whatever comes into your mind. (For example: 'I'm so angry. You really, really piss me off. I'm so jealous of you. Why did you do that to me? It's not fair. It's not my fault. You never listen to me') speak out loud whatever is on your mind. Imagine your little mini-you is having a tantrum and getting it all off her chest. Clenching your fists can be helpful too

   b.   Get a cushion or a pillow and beat it with your fists (or with a tennis racquet or baseball bat if you have one handy) as you express what you are feeling. Say whatever comes into your mind

   c.   Get a small hand towel and wring it tightly as you say aloud exactly what you feel

   d.   Go outside somewhere where there is no-one around: on a beach, in the woods, in a field, or in your car with closed windows – and shout and scream loudly what you feel you want to say – making fists as you do this works wonders

2.   Whatever method you choose, don't hold back. Stamp, beat, shout, wring and say what you need to say until you sense the release and the relief as you let go. This experiment often brings tears to the surface when the anger has faded so accept that and let them flow

3.   It can be an unnerving experience to let go so treat yourself kindly. After your release session, sit quietly, wrap a blanket around yourself and have a warm drink if you feel that would be just perfect

A note if you think this is all a bit scary. I remember an old lady I used to know telling me that it was very common in the 'old days' for women to use making bread every morning as a kind of emotional release. They would beat and pummel the dough strongly as they cursed, fumed, and complained about their husbands, kids, housework, mothers and anything else they had on their mind and wanted to get off their chest and she said they always felt so much better afterwards. Sometimes a group of women would gather around a big kitchen table and all join in as they beat the shit out of their lumps of dough. What a powerhouse kitchen that must have been. And, my old lady friend said, that bread seemed to rise so much bigger and taste so much better for some reason! So, you can rest assured, these emotional release methods are nothing new or revolutionary. Women have been doing something similar for aeons.

Remember whatever happens, speak kindly to yourself and to your little mini-you. She is always there and always listening. Let her be your guiding light as you congratulate yourself for taking care of her and being bold, brave and committed to cracking your code.

CHAPTER 5 KEY POINTS

- Food isn't magic. It cannot make feelings disappear
- Conflicting thoughts confuse your mind. The mind cannot process conflicting thoughts – they cancel each other out and you end up feeling stuck
- Feelings are simply mental and physical messengers trying to tell you to pay attention to something
- Feelings don't disappear. If you prevent a feeling from surfacing it will appear in some other way
- Feelings are just energy moving. E-motion: energy in motion
- It is safe to express your feelings. Feelings are only destructive if they're forbidden or not allowed
- Feelings are there to be experienced, to be felt – not solved
- Your inner child is a guide and a focus for your best intentions and well-being
- Speak kindly to yourself and your little mini-you. She is always present and always listening
- Celebrate every step. You can't get this wrong

CRACK YOUR CODE

1. Practice Experiment Five: What Would Happen If? Make notes in your journal about your discoveries. If there is someone you want to speak to, pluck up the courage to have that conversation if you feel safe to do so. If it doesn't feel safe, share with a friend, your code-cracking partner, a relative you trust or a group you belong to
2. Practise Experiment Six: Loving Your Mini-You. Stay aware of your promise to her and do your very best to keep it
3. Practice Experiment Seven: Space to Feel What You Feel and commit to setting aside some time each week to repeat this experiment

4. Practice Experiment Eight: Let It Rise and Let It Out
    Express your feelings and get them out. Make some bread
    too if you fancy!
5. Try out some of the optional journaling prompts below – as
    many or as few as you like:
    a. When I take a trip down memory lane, what sayings and
        utterings whizzed around my childhood environment?
        How have they affected the way I think about feelings/
        expressing feelings?
    b. Have I got any conflicting thoughts and beliefs? If so,
        what are they how could they be impeding my progress?
    c. How do I feel about loving my mini-me? Do I believe
        she's real?
6. If you have a code cracking partner, share anything you
    choose to with them and listen to them in return. Please be
    supportive and non-judgemental
7. Listen to your self-hypnosis recording: The Quantum Jump
    once each day or evening or just before sleeping (the choice
    is yours), until you have listened to it at least 21 times. If you
    fall asleep that's fine
8. Treat yourself with kindness and self-compassion. Take a
    walk, have a bath, read a book, watch something funny on
    TV, dance, sing in the kitchen, bake some bread, have a chat
    with a friend – anything that fills you with good feelings

When you are ready, move on to the next chapter and start cracking
your emotional weight codes

6

SECONDARY GAINS

Could your weight be doing you a favour?

By now, I hope you understand that food is not your problem – it's what you have been using food for that's the problem. That's why diets will never work to crack compulsive eating codes – because they are all about the food! Restricting it, managing it, controlling it but never getting to the root of why you are eating dry cornflakes straight out the packet at midnight feeling like a failure and vowing to get back on the diet in the morning – again!

As you crack your codes and repeat your experiments, you will safely and in a timely manner, gradually gain confidence in your ability to feel, express and let go. As you face up to your feelings you will find it easier and easier to stop stuffing them down with food and you may begin to release some weight as a bonus result too. However, there is another crucial factor in the equation, a kind of in-tandem process going on because the weight has a function too and unless you also crack that coding, arriving at your happy, healthy weight and staying there will either be well-nigh impossible or if you manage to make it, your results won't stick and you'll start to pile it back on again. The weight will return because it is a secondary gain.

SECONDARY GAINS

You may remember back in Chapter One I said all habits have secondary gains – one or more additional advantages that come along with the basic habit. Subconscious spin-offs that run in-sync with the original coding and in the case of compulsive eating, the secondary gain tends to be weight!

Now I know the idea that the unwanted weight you carry could have a purpose, a function, and could be serving you in some way might seem bizarre. When I first heard of this idea, I thought it was crazy. I hated the weight I was carrying. All I wanted to do was get rid of it. No way was it doing me any favours. However, I learned through my experiments that it was, and accepting this truth was the second vital key to releasing it and letting go of it forever.

If you are like I was, your weight problem consumes a great deal of your attention. Someone I spoke to recently told me that when she did the next experiment, she was shocked to discover that worrying about her weight and hating or despising her body took up most of her head space for about 70% of her day.

Your next experiment is an opportunity to notice how much of your headspace is consumed with thinking about food, weight and your body.

EXPERIMENT NINE: ALL-CONSUMING THOUGHTS

You may not realise just how much you think about your weight and/
or hating your body, despising it, or blaming it so in this experiment, I
want you to monitor your thoughts for a day. Simply for the purpose
of clarity, not for judgement.

1.   Choose a day to do this experiment
2.   On your chosen day, set your phone alarm to remind you hourly
     (while you are awake) to stop whatever you are doing and
     check what you are thinking
3.   Make a quick note or record your thoughts on your phone if it
     has anything to do with your weight, and/or how you feel about
     your body
4.   At the end of the day, check back over your notes
5.   How much time has been taken up with thinking about your
     weight and/or your body?
6.   How do you feel about your observations?
7.   Are you delighted, surprised, shocked, disappointed, happy, sad,
     despairing?
8.   Repeat this experiment on another day and tally your results
9.   Are there differences or similarities? If so, what and what could
     be the causes?
10. What purpose could focusing on your body have?

Gloria said,

'I realised my weight had been helping me to avoid certain situations I didn't dare say no to. I don't enjoy noisy parties, visits to the pub or big friends/family gatherings and I was managing to get out of invitations to these kinds of events, while also avoiding upsetting or displeasing people because of how I felt about my weight.

'I never actually turned down an invite, I wasn't bold enough to do that. I just worried about it for days beforehand so by the time the day of the event arrived I was already in a state of anxiety. Then, a few hours before it was time to get ready, I would begin massively overeating and that would absorb all my attention for a while. As I continued to binge, I would begin to feel disgusted with myself. I would berate myself, saying things like, "You're so disgusting. You're a fraud. You're useless. You're a coward. What is wrong with you, what would your friends think if they knew what a disgusting person you are? Look at you, what a fat slob you've turned into. You can't possibly go out looking like this. Everyone will laugh at you – and nothing will fit anyway."

'By this stage, I would be in tears and the mere idea of looking in the mirror, dressing, or doing my hair would be completely overwhelming yet I would still keep eating. Eventually I would begin to feel nauseous from all the food I had shoved down but with that came a sense of relief because now I had a genuine excuse not to go. I was feeling sick and I could honestly call whoever had invited me and say, "I'm so sorry but I can't come. I feel really ill, I think it must be something I've eaten. I can't possibly come like this. I feel awful." Really what I meant was I felt awful because I thought my body looked like shit, I was a fat slob, and didn't deserve to be near other sane human beings.

'The person I called might be disappointed and/or offer sympathy, help or (heaven forbid) to come round, but I always said, "Thanks, but I'll be fine. It's probably just one of those 24-hour things. Anyway, just in case it is a bug, I wouldn't want to pass it on." Job done! Gathering avoided. No further questions asked.

'Unfortunately, there were unpleasant consequences beyond the nausea. My evening alone would then usually involve more eating to soothe my guilt and shame and end with falling into bed in a stuffed stupor. I would wake the next day dreading any friendly phone calls when I would have to lie again. However, in spite of all of that discomfort, my pay-off was I had evaded a dreaded gathering once again.

'I have finally understood that my eating and my weight have saved me hundreds of times from saying I didn't want to go to some event or upset people I cared about and now I know I have choices. If I want anything to change, I must do and say things that my body had been saying and doing for me. Then the weight and the eating that caused it can let go. I won't need it any more.'

With these insights, Gloria took some big, bold steps. She plucked up the courage to talk to her friends and family and tell them she didn't like going to parties and noisy places. She didn't tell them what she had been doing to avoid them. That was too difficult and not necessary. All she needed to say was the truth – which was that she wasn't a party pooper or unsociable, she was simply a quiet soul who loved seeing and meeting people in quiet places or small groups because crowds and noise made her feel anxious and overwhelmed. So, in future could they meet like that? Unsurprisingly, everyone said of course and organised new ways of meeting. Gloria also dared to invite small groups of people to her home and never once did she binge beforehand or try to get out of it.

With an open mind and further investigation, she discovered that her weight had been doing many other things for her too and one by one she took over each role consciously. And the more she did that, the easier and easier it became to stop eating compulsively and to let the weight go naturally.

HOW YOUR WEIGHT COULD BE SUBCONSIOUSLY DOING YOU A FAVOUR

Remember, our mind is genetically programmed to move toward pleasure and away from pain. Even though any unwanted weight you're carrying may be a painful experience for you, your mind is hanging onto it for some reason. The weight has a role, a function, a purpose in your life. It is what I call emotional weight or emotional padding. When you accept the possibility there may be a positive intention (or more than one) underneath it and become curious without judging yourself, you open an opportunity to crack your 'hang on to my weight' codes. Below are some of the ways your weight may be helping you out:

- Obsessing about your body and your weight may divert you from dealing with your feelings. You focus on the weight and how you feel about it, rather than what's causing you to eat compulsively in the first place
- Your weight may be insulating you against the outside world, acting as a buffer zone
- Your weight may be providing an excuse to not do certain things when you don't have the courage to speak up and say what you do or don't want
- Your weight may be saying 'No' when you don't dare to
- Your weight may be a big 'Fuck you' to a society that celebrates thinness
- Your weight could be trying to send out signals in the hope that someone will get the message, such as: I'm distressed, unhappy, don't feel good about myself, don't care for myself, please help me
- Your weight could be bringing you attention, sympathy, help, support that you don't dare to ask for in case you don't get it
- Your weight may be helping you to hide in situations you find challenging
- You may have the belief that overweight is overlooked so your weight helps you to deflect unwanted attention

- You may be scared or wary of sexual advances and believe being bigger will keep potential admirers away
- Your weight may be your inner rebel showing up
- You believe 'you can't have it all' – if you are otherwise successful and fulfilled this is the one thing that you can't crack that proves your belief
- Your weight allows you to be part of a club, group, family group of like bodied people. It gives you a sense of connection and belonging
- Hanging on to your weight ensures you don't have to deal with jealousy from your friends or family who are unsuccessfully trying to shed weight
- You have a belief that you are unworthy, not enough, you don't deserve to be happy in your skin and your body demonstrates that for you
- You believe slim equates with worth and happiness and as you also have a belief that you are unworthy, not enough, don't deserve to be happy in your skin, your body demonstrates and confirms these beliefs
- You secretly think it's vain to want to look great, feel great, be healthy and happy in your body so heaven forbid anyone else would think that about you

It is common to have more than one subconscious weight code running and serving different hidden purposes, just as you have discovered often happens with your eating behaviour. When we interlink the two components – compulsive eating and consequent weight gain – we have complex interconnecting codes creating an intricate web of results all working in harmony as our subconscious mind does its job of moving us away from pain and towards pleasure. Now I know you are probably thinking: 'Well, these codes can't be working as I'm certainly not noticing any pleasure here', but your coding has been serving you somehow and until you are clear about why you've been accumulating and hanging on to weight, you will be stuck in your wanting-to-shed-it-but-never-letting-it-go loop forever.

The following experiment will help you decode this dilemma.

EXPERIMENT TEN: IS MY WEIGHT SERVING ME?

This experiment is a non-judgmental way of decoding possible subconscious functions and intentions of any emotional weight you are carrying. Get a cup of something satisfying, have your pen and journal ready, be comfortable and relax. Take your time and just allow your answers to bubble up. Be as honest as you can in your responses. No-one need ever know what you write unless you choose to tell them. This experiment is for you and your awareness.

1. Name the issue, problem, dilemma etc., e.g.: I have a lot of weight I don't want on my body, or I hate my fat, or I feel embarrassed/ashamed about how much I weight, I am sick of being overweight, I keep getting fatter etc. Describe your problem in a way that has meaning for you, use your words.
2. Now answer these three questions:
   a. What does having this problem/issue/dilemma prevent me from being in my life?
   b. What does having this problem/issue/dilemma prevent me from doing in my life?
   c. What does this having problem/issue/dilemma prevent me from having in my life?
3. Now answer these three questions:
   a. What does having this problem/issue/dilemma allow me to be in my life?
   b. What does having this problem/issue/dilemma allow me to do in my life?
   c. What does this having problem/issue/dilemma allow me to have in my life?
4. Now answer these questions:
   a. What do I need to do/not do or say/not say to begin to make the changes I want to make?
   b. What is challenging for me about that?
5. Be grateful. Your body and your mind have been helping you out of situations you thought or think you can't handle

6. Say this (aloud or inside your head), 'Part of me that has been helping me out all these years, I am deeply thankful. You have protected me in so many ways but now I am ready and willing to consciously take on your roles and tasks for myself so you can let go now. I am ready to release you now'
7. Finally answer this question:
    a. What am I **willing** to do or say in the next seven days to consciously take on at least one of the tasks my weight has kindly been doing for me? Write that down in your journal now.
8. Commit to doing that and begin the release. More actions will bring more release

Janice was molested at a party even though she felt sure her size would keep any man away from her. She was standing quietly in the corner by herself when a man came up behind her and just grabbed her bottom. She felt shocked, angry and upset all at once, but she just swallowed her feelings and moved away from him. The man followed her across the room, so she went into the kitchen. He followed her there smiling and still trying to touch her, asking if she was playing hard to get. It was only when she let her fury at being ignored and abused rise and finally shouted 'Get your grubby little hands off me right now you pervert' in front of all the people at the party, that the man stopped his nasty game. He rapidly left the party, slinking out the door in embarrassment. She was immediately applauded and celebrated by her friends for standing up for herself and from then on, she dared to let her feelings out more and more. She began to claim her space and create clear boundaries with her voice and her actions rather than trying to give out smoke signals with her body that not everyone could or wanted to interpret. Janice noticed the more she stood up for herself, saying no to people, things, events, situations she was no longer prepared to tolerate in her life the less she was driven to eat compulsively.

You can't hate yourself thin. You've might have tried that, but it doesn't work. However, an attitude of gratitude, being grateful to your problems, seeing them as gifts that have been trying to help you move away from pain, get you out of difficulties, maybe in some extreme cases even saving your life, can work wonders. Try it.

SEX, SMOKE SIGNALS AND BOUNDARIES

Over my years of working with women with eating and weight problems, the issues of sex and boundaries often crop up. Many women – but not all so this section may not apply to you – have realised that being bigger has been a subconscious attempt to deflect unwanted sexual attention and advances without having to open their mouths. This may have worked for some women but there are always people who find a bigger body very attractive and a thinner one less so, so it's not an ideal solution. We may think we are signalling 'Stay away from me/I'm unattractive/I'm not into sex/I don't like you/Fuck off and leave me alone' via our bodies but our signals might not be received as we intend. And, even if they are, success doesn't necessarily follow. The solution lies of course in opening your mouth to speak, to dare to say what you want to say and express what you really feel rather than to shove food down to bury the anger, resentment or despair you may feel at being or feeling vulnerable.

SAYING 'NO'

When we can say no to things outside of ourselves, the easier it becomes to say no to food when we are not hungry.

Important safety clause: if you find yourself in a situation where your safety is at risk in any way, this is not the time to claim your boundaries unless you are highly skilled in self-defence – even then, your first job is to get to a place of safety if you can and to get or call for help. Personal safety is your number one job – you can deal with your boundaries later.

Remember as you decipher your weight and body codes, keep an attitude of gratitude. Your body has been helping you and trying to stand up for you when you found it difficult or impossible to do so at the time. As always, speak kindly to yourself and appreciate how brave you are as you allow the real, authentic you to emerge from behind the shields of compulsive eating and emotional weight.

CHAPTER 6 KEY POINTS

- Your weight could be doing you a favour – even though you hate it
- There are potential secondary gains from hanging on to weight
- Obsessing about your weight may take up a large percentage of your thinking time and divert you away from feeling and/ addressing what you really need to feel and address
- The subconscious codes of compulsive eating and weight accumulation are complex and interlinked
- To release secondary gain weight for good, you must be willing to take on its roles, functions and intentions consciously. Nothing changes until you take action
- Be grateful to your weight before and as you release it
- Speak kindly to yourself. Celebrate every step. You can't get this wrong

CRACK YOUR CODE

1. Practice Experiment Nine: All-Consuming Thoughts.
    Choose an additional day and monitor your thinking. What
    percentage of this day is taken up by worrying about your
    weight and your body? What are your thoughts on that
    result? Are you surprised?
2. Practice Experiment Ten: Is My Weight Serving Me? Take
    your time. Take days over this experiment if you want to.
    Be as honest and open as you can to discovering interesting
    things about yourself and how your weight may be helping
    or hindering what you want to be, do, and have in your life.
    Be non-judgemental and self-accepting
3. If there is someone you want to speak to, and/or actions
    you want to take, pluck up the courage to have those
    conversations and to do those things if you feel safe. If it
    doesn't feel safe, share with a friend, your code-cracking
    partner, a relative you trust or a group you belong to
4. If you have a code cracking partner share anything you
    choose to and listen to them in return. Please be supportive
    and non-judgemental
5. Continue to listen to your self-hypnosis recording: The
    Quantum Jump. You know the mind learns by repetition and
    you can always learn more
6. Treat yourself with kindness and self-compassion. Take a
    walk, have a bath, read a book, watch something funny on
    TV, dance, sing in the kitchen, bake some bread, have a chat
    with a friend – anything that fills you with good feelings

When you are ready, move on to the next chapter and start
reprogramming your mind to maintain your healthy weight forever!

SELF REGULATION

The Great Refresh

Every baby is born knowing instinctively when they are hungry and when they are full. If you've ever kept a tiny baby waiting to be fed you will know how it doesn't take long before their cries get louder, and their desperation grows. However, as soon as the breast or the bottle reaches their little mouth they begin to calm down, feel soothed very quickly and relax. And, if you've ever tried to overfeed a tiny baby you will also know how difficult that can be. When they are full, the baby will turn away, close their mouth firmly, or vomit up anything that is too much for them. We are born with natural hunger and fulness cues encoded into our brains and they never leave us. We may learn to override them or deny them for all manner of reasons, but they are always there, ready and waiting for us to tune back in and take advantage of our natural body intelligence. Learning how to trust and follow your natural body cues again, allowing your original coding to perform its natural function is, in my personal and professional experience, one of the most effective routes out of compulsive eating, binge eating, weight and body obsession, endless dieting failures and all the accompanying despair and distress that comes along with these states. It is also the most physically and mentally satisfying way to come to and maintain your natural healthy weight forever.

Now, I know how scary or ridiculous the idea of trusting your body can be when you have been battling with it for years. My initial reaction to the idea when my therapist first told me about it was 'Well that won't work for me. I have no idea what it feels like to be hungry or full any more' and I've heard many women over the years say exactly the same. However, by the time I had arrived at this stage of my food freedom journey, and after so many experiments that had proved I was onto something that could change my life forever,

I decided to trust my therapist's experience and give tuning into my natural cues a go. She reminded me that I didn't have to believe what she was saying, she wasn't asking me to believe anything. All she asked was that I suspend my disbelief for a while, practice the experiments she gave me, and draw my own conclusions.

I was so scared. Scared of getting fatter, scared of losing control, scared of failing, scared of feeling disappointed again, scared that all the changes I had already made would go out the window if I dared to jump into this forgotten way of being. Then I realised that was the key. I had simply forgotten how to live by my natural coding, I had overwritten it in various ways, but it was still there patiently waiting for my attention. It was my birthright and I could re-learn how to use it and see what happened. I decided it was time to let go and trust. I began with challenging my persistent diet mentality, my food rules and my addiction to constantly weighing myself and this is how you take your first steps into remembering and tuning in to your birth right too.

DITCH THE DIET

It isn't easy to release ourselves from the grip of dieting. Dieting and controlling what we allow ourselves to eat seem to offer the perfect fix for our eating and weight problems. Almost all the medical advice, one way or another, takes this apparently logical approach and of course the diet industry tells us it's true – they are an industry after all and their goal is profit, not your health and well-being whatever their advertising blurb might say.

However, as we know, the diet solution rarely works long term, or even for very long at all; statistics show that 95% of people who go on a diet may lose weight but they will most likely regain it, and maybe even more, within about five years. So, are you ready to take a risk? To experiment with the idea of ditching dieting? To try something different as you have proof – and probably plenty of it – that what you have been doing, for however long you've been doing it, hasn't been working?

NO FOOD RULES

No food is inherently bad or evil even though some slimming regimes – and I'm naming no names here but I think you might know who I mean – allow you some 'sins' if you've been 'good'! Labelling food as good or bad or telling yourself, and maybe others, that you have been good or bad because you have or haven't eaten something on or off your permitted list isn't helpful and triggers stress. If we've had a good day, we worry about if we will be able to keep it going. If we've had a bad day, we chastise ourselves for having given in to our desires and feel guilty, weak and ashamed. Stressing and worrying about food and eating is not motivating and in fact the hormone cortisol, which is released by the adrenal glands when we are in stress mode, can leads to us storing fat especially around the mid-line. Worrying about food and being fat increases fat. Anxiety about weight loss can sometimes cause you to gain weight not shed it. So, from now on, no food is out of bounds, no food is off limits, no food is forbidden. Food is neutral.

However, there is one proviso here. Even though there are no good or bad foods per se, some foods in our modern world are so packed full of chemicals and additives that they are almost non-foods. As you experiment with breaking free from your food rules, for the sake of your health and well-being I encourage you to avoid foods that start from a chemical base as much as possible and if it's financially viable for you. Chocolate, sausages, cheeses, biscuits, pasta, cakes, meats, cereals, bread, cream, ice cream etc., made from real ingredients are all fine and if expense is a challenge, go for real as much as you can. Now this doesn't mean you never eat junk food or industrially produced food but you prioritise real food over non-food most of the time.

Please Note: I'm not suggesting that if you have a health condition that requires certain food choices, or if you have certain ethical or religious reasons for avoiding particular foods or food groups you should cast all that to the winds, no. You can allow your natural cues to guide your choices within your personal health paradigm and trust your mind and body to align with that.

No food rules also means there are no right times or wrong times to eat. No rules about eating three meals a day or not snacking between meals. No rules about not eating after a certain time in the evening. All that is off the menu along with calorie counting, macros, fasting, carbs are good or bad, avoid all fats, never eat more than three pieces of fruit a day. The lists of limits and restrictions we are advised to stick to are never ending and ever changing and they are all working against you being a free human with the ability to naturally self-regulate your eating.

Attention: look out for the food police! All of us who have struggled with dieting, weight, compulsive eating and body shame have an inner Food Cop giving us strict instructions about what we should and shouldn't eat and why. If you listen, she is probably yelling and waving her truncheon right now. She might be saying 'Don't listen to this rubbish. You know you're weak and there's no way you could ever trust your body. You'll be as fat as a pig in no time if you eat what you want' or perhaps 'This Charya woman, what does she know? Food is neutral? What crap. She's obviously a nutter. Don't listen to her. You just need to be stricter with yourself, have stronger will-power, you need to stay on a diet forever, get back behind the restrictions line, it makes sense' and so she goes on and on. It can help if you realise that she is just a habit, a code, she is not real and she is not 'you'. She is a self-protection device you subconsciously installed sometime in your past, but you don't have to believe her. She may have helped you out a million times, making you feel safe as you tried to stick to her instructions and you can be grateful for that, but if you keep letting her direct your every food and eating move you will keep suffering. So, when your Food Cop bangs on your door, and she will I assure you, you just say 'I didn't call you. There's no crime here and you can go away right now'. Each time you do that, you overwrite your cop code and create a new, refreshed conscious code of food freedom. However, be aware. Your Food Cop can hang around for years and it may take long-term consistent and insistent statements of 'I didn't call you and there's no crime here' to calm her down and eventually get her to give up. But that's okay. Every knock on your door is another opportunity to refresh and consolidate your conscious food freedom code.

DON'T MAKE RULES OUT OF NO RULES!

Finally, don't turn this way of eating into another diet regime! Don't make rules out of the no rules approach and then beat yourself up for not sticking to it. There is no wagon to fall off. You are experimenting and there will be challenges for sure, but perfection is not part of the game. Try out everything and congratulate yourself for every single shift you make. No-one I have ever met, or read about, or heard of sticks to the no rules approach all the time as life is complicated and perfection is no fun anyway.

Please note: what follows on the next pages is a comprehensive set of experiments. Experiments Ten through to Thirteen can be done in sync as you will see but they don't have to be. If you prefer to spread them out, that's fine. However, Experiment Eleven is fundamental so start there regardless of how else you choose to go through this chapter, okay?

EXPERIMENT ELEVEN: EAT WHEN YOU'RE HUNGRY, STOP WHEN YOU'RE FULL

It is particularly important to be patient with yourself in this experiment. Knowing when to start eating and when to stop isn't generally easy to gauge if you have been using food to try to help deal with life's challenges. However, I assure you with time and practice you can gradually refresh your hunger and fullness cues and learn to trust your body again but even then, it may not always be possible some of the time. Family, economic, work, living situations and various other circumstances might make it complicated so do whatever you can within your personal life and lifestyle and always remember, perfection is impossible. Go easy on yourself. You can't get this wrong, okay? It's an experiment and there are no right answers, just potential discoveries personal to you. Read through both parts of the experiment first and use them side by side for seven days.

PART ONE: EAT WHEN YOU'RE HUNGRY

1. First, choose a day to start and write that date in your journal so it is recorded and you are self-accountable
2. From that date, for seven consecutive days whenever you think of eating, or the idea crosses your mind, take a breath and pause for a few moments or minutes before you start eating
3. In these moments, ask yourself 'Am I really hungry? What do I feel as I wait? Do I have any sensations in my stomach, is there a gentle rumbling or sense of light emptiness? Are there any sensations in my mouth, or anywhere else in my body?'
4. If the answer to any or some of your questions is yes, then go on to ask yourself 'What do I really want? Do I want something crunchy, smooth, hot, cold, sharp, sweet?' and be as specific as you can. Then, allow yourself to eat just what comes to you. Remember there are No Food Rules! Give yourself permission to eat anything you choose to eat even though it may be challenging everything you have come to believe
5. Special Tip: Try not to wait until you hunger is intense as that tends to drive you to eat as soon as possible and not allow for

tuning in to the subtleties of what might satisfy you. As soon as you sense what I call a whisper of hunger, pause and begin to ask the questions about what you really want

6.   This process will help you to not only begin to refresh your cues it will also start building self-trust because you are willing to give yourself just what you genuinely want, when you genuinely want it

7.   If after your self-questions you realise you are not hungry after all, congratulate yourself for the awareness you now have and see if you can wait until you *are* hungry and if you can then eat what you really want

PART TWO: STOP WHEN YOU ARE FULL

Sensing fullness can be equally as difficult to recognise as hunger. How does it feel to be comfortably full, satisfied, satiated? Again, taking a pause can really help.

1.   During your seven days, when you are eating, whether you realise you're just eating mindlessly or you've chosen what you want to eat when you want it, at some point before you finish whatever it is, take a breath and pause

2.   Take a little rest from eating and check in to see if you really do want to continue or if you've had enough for now. If after your pause you decide to continue, go ahead and eat mindfully if possible (see the slow down practice that follows). If not, stop and check back in about twenty minutes and if you are still interested in your food, eat it and enjoy it

3.   Notice the 'phew'. This is something Sarah, a group member said when we were sharing our experiences of how to recognise fullness and I found it so descriptive and useful I'm passing it on. She said, 'When I'm full I always seem to say 'phew' so I've made that my signal to stop eating'.

Since Sarah shared that wonderful bit of advice, I've noticed many people spontaneously doing the 'phew' thing quite instinctively so you could test it out and see if it works for you.

Make notes in your journal as you go through your seven days.

SOME POSSIBLE CHALLENGES THAT MAY ARISE

- Certain times are more challenging than others
- You find it difficult to sense when you are hungry or full
- This all seems impossible in your work/family/living/financial situation
- You encounter strong feelings when you wait to eat or feel full
- Strong, counter beliefs come up
- People question you and what you are doing
- It's all just too much!

SOME POTENTIAL SOLUTIONS

- First, accept that no-one ever, EVER, gets it right or sorted from the start. Refreshing back to your natural coding takes time, patience and tolerance. You are challenging your own learned coding and family, cultural and social beliefs, diet culture, medical opinion, the latest food fads from influencers on Instagram, maybe general nutritional guidelines – the list is long so give yourself a break and do whatever you can when you can. Every positive step takes you closer to embodying that gorgeous, free, confident, healthy, happy in her skin woman you dream of being
- Be curious about why certain times are more challenging. What's going on at those times? Who are you with or are you alone? What time of day/evening/night is it? Are you sticking to fixed times of eating even if you are not hungry? Are you still in diet mode perhaps as this will make this experiment more difficult?
- Allow yourself time. Noticing your cues may take a while. Be patient and stay aware. They will become apparent with awareness. It takes time, consistency and repetition to let go of old codes that don't serve you any more and to retune and refresh your natural ones
- If work schedules make it difficult to flow with your hunger/

fullness cues do your best to at least have food you love, that tastes great, that is free from limits. You can still notice when you are hungry and full. And, outside of work hours, practice this experiment

- If your family situation means that you eat with others at certain times, perhaps you can have at least one or two meals or snacks each day when you do your own thing. If you have been/are a compulsive eater I'm certain you've managed to eat outside of designated times a number of times before! And remember, just because your cultural/family/social conditioning dictates a certain set of rules about when to eat, and maybe also what's acceptable to eat at those times that doesn't mean it has to be that way. Flexibility might work for other people that haven't ever considered it too

- If financial constraints seem to get in the way of having a variety food available that your body genuinely wants, again do your best within the limits of what is possible. Whatever our situation, we can always ask ourselves the basic sets of questions: The 'Am I really hungry?' set and the 'Am I full?' set. They are the fundamentals. The crucial code cracking questions and you can work around the rest. Remember, the mind's number one job is to move us away from pain and towards pleasure and it will try any ruse to do that. Don't allow finances to get in the way of your natural instincts – be creative and overwrite your self-protection codes and refresh your original ones

- As you practice this experiment, it's inevitable that strong feelings will arise. Don't let that deter you from doing the work. You have a package of resources in Chapters Five and Six so use them to help you over and through any emotional barriers that crop up

- Deeply entrenched beliefs about what/when/where/how/how much we are supposed to eat will likely also crop up. Many women I have worked with are knocked of course by the old favourite 'You must clean your plate because … the kids in Africa are starving, your dad worked hard to buy that food, it's a sin to waste food' or whatever adage was bandied about when you were growing up. Another one is the 'You can't eat that for breakfast/lunch/tea/dinner'. I once had a boyfriend who told me I was childish because I loved eating chocolate cake for breakfast. Needless to say, I vehemently disagreed but he persisted with his limiting beliefs about food and mealtimes. It wasn't long before our relationship was over and I went on eating whatever I wanted, whenever I wanted it! We don't have to believe what we believe or what we think or what others believe or think. Question your beliefs. Overwrite them. Create new ones you prefer. They are all illusions anyway. No belief is the actual 'truth'

- If other people question or criticise what you are doing, you have various options. You can either engage in those conversations or ignore them. You can explain clearly what you are experimenting with and you can ask for help and support. You may be pleasantly surprised by the support you can enlist when you honestly explain what you are doing and why

- If you feel overwhelmed sometimes, it's okay to take a pause. Take a day off. Let it all go. Relax and accept it really doesn't matter. If you lose track for a day or two or more, just get back on track when you are ready. No judgement, no guilt, no beating yourself up. Keep your vision of what you want to be, do, and have in your mind and keep asking yourself the question 'What would she do, what would that woman I want to be do right now?' and you do that

- A relaxed attitude is always the best thing and stress doesn't help us at all

As you eat what you want to eat, when you want to – and at other times when you don't manage to get to that stage – practicing mindful eating regularly is helpful for tuning in to your natural body cues. You can practice the experiment anytime, anywhere

EXPERIMENT TWELVE: MINDFUL EATING

For this experiment, it helps if you sit to eat but it's not essential.

1. When you notice the thought of eating comes to you or you are about to eat, turn off or remove from view as many distractions as possible such as phones, TVs, magazines, books, etc., while you practice this experiment. Sit if that's an option. If not, be still

2. If you haven't already, choose the food you want and have it before you

3. Now stop and before you begin to eat, notice your breathing. Slowing and deepening your breathing increases relaxation. Take five deep breaths

4. Now relax the muscles in your face, drop your shoulders, sink into the chair supporting you or relax as you stand

5. Now look at the food you're about to eat notice the colours, the shapes, the textures, the smell of the food

6. Now begin to eat, chewing slowly. Savour every bite. Whatever it is you eat, taste it, enjoy it. Allow yourself the pleasure of eating

7. As you practise this way of eating it's normal to find your mind wandering, losing focus on the food, the taste, the pleasure, maybe you speed up a little .. when you notice that, just take your mind back to the experience, slow down, breathe, relax and continue as before. Focusing on every morsel, savouring the experience

8. From time to time as you practise mindful eating, apply the pause effect. Take a rest from eating. Look around, notice your relaxation level, your breathing. Come back to eating if you sense you still want more food if not end this experiment and repeat it another time when you eat

What do you enjoy about this experiment? What surprises you? What do you notice? How often do you stop and breathe?

THE CASE OF THE DISAPPEARING TOAST

One breakfast time a while ago, I was practising mindful eating. I prepared a beautiful table with attractive cutlery and crockery and my favourite French strawberry jam. I had two toasted slices of my favourite bread and freshly ground coffee ready to go.

I breathed deeply, I relaxed. It was a beautiful morning. The sun was shining into my kitchen. I felt so good, so in the moment. I opened the jam and smelled the sweet strawberries. As I pushed down the plunger of my coffee pot, the smell of the coffee tickled my nose and I listened to the sound of the coffee pouring into my cute glass coffee cup. I felt the cold stainless steel of the knife and listened to the sound of its scraping as I spread some jam on the first slice of toast. Halfway through that slice, I took a break, put the toast down, drank some coffee. Wonderful. I looked at my sunny garden for a few moments and then returned to the toast and finished the first slice.

What happened next was a vivid reminder of how mindful eating is an ongoing practice! Out of the blue my phone rang. Normally I wouldn't have my phone near me when I practise mindful eating but for some reason I'd forgotten to put it to one side. I automatically reached out, put it on speaker mode and engaged in a conversation for about 10 minutes. When the conversation was over, I looked at my plate and there was no toast. I knew I'd only eaten one slice – but the second one had vanished.

I got up from my chair and looked under the table, under the chair. I was completely convinced I must have dropped it on the floor, but it was nowhere to be seen. I was baffled. Then it struck me. I must have spread jam on that second slice and mindlessly eaten it while talking on the phone. It was as if it hadn't happened, but I learned a valuable lesson. The case of the disappearing toast was the most vivid example I've ever experienced about the effects of being unaware of what we are eating. You see, when I finished talking, I wanted another piece of toast because it felt like I hadn't eaten that second slice at all. I felt empty and unsatisfied because the memory of eating it didn't seem to register in me physically or mentally.

I made more toast and more coffee and I ended up eating three slices instead of my intended two. Which was fine of course. No judgment or guilt, right? Nothing serious had happened. In fact, I found it funny but I know when I was in my restricted-eating previous life such a mishap would have caused me stress for the rest of the day. It might have triggered a binge eating episode or tripped me into limiting food for days to mask the guilt and hopelessness I would have felt after falling off my perfection wagon.

I told my vanishing toast story to all my friends. I even posted about it on Instagram and Facebook because I found it so hilarious and such a great lesson for me. The lesson wasn't just how unaware I was at that time but also that mindful eating, slow, aware eating is an ongoing practice and there's always something to learn whether we are aware or not.

There is no right way to do any of the experiments in this book as lessons can be learned in everything we do and everything we don't. Relaxation, self-acceptance and patience are vital keys to your success – and if you don't always manage these attitudes that's absolutely fine too. Remember we're not going for perfection we're going for progress.

Eating alone, your next experiment, is a great way to bring your attention to how, when and what you eat, and to your hunger and fullness cues.

EXPERIMENT THIRTEEN: EAT ALONE

1. At least once each day, (if that's too difficult for you to arrange, go for every other day) eat alone with no distractions. No TV, phone, book, magazine, laptop, radio etc. It doesn't have to be a full meal; a snack of any kind will do. (I have practiced this experiment with a single biscuit, in a café with coffee and cake, on a park bench eating apples, at my table with a three-course meal)
2. Sit. Preferably at a table but any seat will do. Whatever you eat, eat slowly and mindfully, remembering to breathe and to pause now and then
3. Notice how you feel. Treasure these moments in time and space

How easy it is to create time alone? If it's not easy, what situations could you create that would allow you to practise this experiment? Who do you think will be most affected if you choose to eat alone sometimes?

The next experiment is one of my favourites!

EXPERIMENT FOURTEEN: SCRAPE IT, TIP IT, OR DROP IT!

1. Every time you eat a meal or enjoy a snack, scrape, drop or tip something into the bin. A spoonful or a few crumbs will do. The amount isn't important
2. As you scrape, drop or tip the food, notice any voices whispering in your ear – if there are voices, whose are they? What are they saying?
3. How do you feel? What are you thinking? How easy or difficult is this experiment?

When I suggest this experiment to women I work with, what appears to be simple and easy often turns out to be one of the most challenging to try. All manner of beliefs and codes block their ability to leave some food, even if they're not hungry. 'You must eat everything up on your plate, think of the starving children in Africa, it's a sin to waste food, (my mother's favourite), we haven't got money to burn, your father worked hard for the money to buy that food' are some of the encoded beliefs running their personal eating programmes. I'm sure some are familiar to you, and you may have others of your own. These codes are so compelling that I have seen women break down in tears over their inability to scrape just one teaspoonful of peas into the bin.

This is such a great experiment for exposing how powerful these ingrained codes can be and how difficult it can be to challenge them. As adult women my clients all know consciously that these rules are nonsensical but wow, how subconsciously persuasive this nonsense can be. If these ideas are programmed into you when you are young by someone significant, with an added sprinkling of emotional charge that implies something bad will happen or you will upset someone you love if you don't finish everything on your plate, a strong urge is created to finish up the lot. Even though that coding may have been installed years ago, it is still running – and it will keep on running until you expose it, question it, eradicate it and install coding you want about your adult relationship with food, eating, and your body.

The Scrape It, Tip It, Or Drop It! experiment is brilliant in its simplicity because by taking one small, regular action, you create multiple effects. Each time you leave some food or toss it in the bin, you are erasing those old codes and creating new ones. You are communicating to your mind that you can say no to food, you can stop when you're full, you will decide how much you want to eat and that you are no longer influenced by other people's ideas and beliefs. You are consciously choosing to create a new, adult code relevant your life now. Leaving food is no longer an emotional event that potentially summons up feelings of guilt, fear or any number of other illogical reactive states it's just simply a preference, a choice, something you can do or not with no emotional charge attached.

In hypnosis, Syrena went back to a scene in her early childhood where her father was making her sit at the table until she finished whatever was given to her, even if she didn't like the food, even if it had become cold. This happened quite often she recalled. Her father was a frightening figure, a bully. If she disobeyed him at the table, sometimes he hit her and in her little mind not finishing food became subconsciously connected to pain and fear. That subconscious code continued to run until she examined it as an adult and gained a new perspective. In her hypnosis session, she eventually talked to her father as if he was there with her saying, 'I'm not scared of you now, I am not a tiny frightened little girl. You can't bully me any more. That little girl isn't me now. I'm not four. I'm a strong, adult woman. I'm sixty-seven years old and enough is enough. I can choose what to eat and how much to eat so fuck off and leave me alone'.

Afterwards, Syrena said 'Going back like that made me realise I have been stuck as a little girl who is still scared of her daddy bullying her and hitting her – even though he has been dead for years. I understand now why it's been so hard to leave food. It all makes sense. I knew rationally he couldn't hurt me any more, but I didn't realise how strong and long lasting the impact of those experiences was. I didn't get it that the coding was still running all these years later. I just knew I would feel overwhelmed at the idea of not clearing my plate'.

With that new learning, Syrena took back her power. At the age of sixty-seven, she began to take care of that little girl inside and herself as an adult. She ate what she loved when she was hungry and stopped when she was full – however much was left on her plate – and frequently tuned into her mini-me to make sure she was satisfied too. She scraped something in the bin every time she ate and gradually, through repeating this simple action over and over she built a new code of freedom and choice after years and years of confusion and pain.

Your next experiment takes you travelling to France — well, in attitude at least!

EXPERIMENT FIFTEEN: BE LIKE THE FRENCH

Starting right this minute, be like the French. From this moment on, honour food and eating.

1. Buy and eat the best kind of food you can afford
2. If you want chocolate, cheese, bread, biscuits, cake, vegetables, meat, fish, fruit, eggs, pasta, rice, vegetarian or vegan, take away or restaurant food, whatever you want, have the best quality that fits within your budget
3. Create a sense of occasion and elegance around your eating. If you are eating at home, set the table well. Use your best cutlery and crockery don't save it up for special occasions. Make every eating experience a special occasion
4. Add a vase flowers or candles sometimes and sit somewhere with a pleasant view if you can
5. Take your time. Relax, relish and enjoy every morsel, every moment – and remember, the more you relax and breathe, the easier you process and digest your food and the more likely you are to notice what you genuinely want and when you are genuinely full. Value and honour each bite
6. Be like the French who are renowned for taking hours over lunch and see what happens

CHAPTER 7 KEY POINTS

- You were born with natural hunger and fullness cues encoded into your brain. You may have learned to override them or deny them, but they are always there
- No food is inherently good or bad. Food is neutral
- Dieting doesn't work long term for most people and may cause your weight to increase
- Don't make rules out of the no rules process
- Slowing down to eat gives you the greatest opportunity to tune into your natural hunger and fullness cues
- Bring awareness to your eating. Be like the French. Honour food and eating
- Speak kindly to yourself. Celebrate every step. You can't get this wrong

CRACK YOUR CODE

1. Practice Experiment Eleven: Eat When You're Hungry, Stop When You're Full. Be patient and compassionate with yourself in this experiment. After seven days, keep going day after day until noticing and responding to your natural cues becomes your automatic code again
2. Check out the possible challenges you may encounter during Experiment Eleven and the potential solutions
3. Practice Experiment Twelve: Mindful Eating and Experiment Thirteen: Eat Alone. Notice how bringing your awareness to eating affects you. Practice them together sometimes
4. Practice Experiment Fourteen: Scrape It, Tip It, or Drop It! Create a habit of leaving a little food each time you eat by doing it regularly. The mind learns by repetition
5. Step into French mode regularly and notice the effect

6. If difficult feelings arise at any time, refer to the Feelings Chapter for suggestions on how to release them. If unpleasant memories return, if you wish to speak to anyone about them and you think they will listen and accept what you want to say, do so. Enlist help and support from a friend or relative if you need it. Or, if you prefer, write a letter you will never send to anyone concerned and lay everything out on the table. Get it all out on paper and then burn it or throw it away

7. Try out some of the optional journaling prompts below – as many or as few as you like:

    a. What beliefs did I expose when I practiced Scrape It, Tip It, or Drop It?

    b. Am I still in diet mode? If so, what scares me about dropping it?

8. If you have a code cracking partner, share anything you choose to and listen to them in return

9. Continue to listen to your self-hypnosis recording: The Quantum Jump. You know the mind learns by repetition and there is always more to learn

10. Treat yourself with loving kindness and honour your body every day

When you are ready, move on to the next chapter: Food Freedom: Your New Code

8

FOOD FREEDOM: YOUR NEW CODE

The incredible lightness of being

Like almost everyone who comes to me for help with their eating and weight issues, the primary motivating factor that induced you to pick up this book was probably your desire to lose weight. You still believed that losing weight was the answer to your prayers and maybe my system would do the trick finally and forever. I hope you now understand it's not that simple!

To get to a place where we feel happy in our skin and our lives are not ruled by food, body obsession, dieting and repeatedly jumping on and falling off wagons, we need to understand that it's not about the food. It's about so much more. It's about cracking our compulsive eating codes, expressing our emotions, changing our behaviour and our thinking, and consciously taking on the roles and tasks that our weight has been subconsciously performing for us. It's about understanding that each time we change or overwrite one tiny bit of our previous coding we are reprogramming our mind and installing new codes of self-trust, resilience, emotional strength, authenticity and self-awareness. And, as we release the need to eat over our feelings our physical, 'emotional weight' can release too. Slowly and gently the body can let go and come to its happy, healthy weight and settle there without effort, stress, limits or restrictions. When that happens, we can trust that we have reprogrammed our mind to maintain our happy weight forever.

SET POINT THEORY: WHAT IS YOUR HAPPY WEIGHT?

People come in all shapes and sizes and your natural, or what I call your 'happy' weight, is an individual, balanced, harmonised state that is biologically and uniquely right for you. This is known as your 'set point'. A weight where your body is comfortable and settles without stress, effort, struggle or restrictions. The term is a little misleading as it is in fact a range, a kind of biological comfort zone with the purpose of keeping you within about ten pounds of your natural weight depending on your metabolism and body state. This so-called set point works somewhat like a thermostat but instead of maintaining a steady temperature, it is constantly adjusting to try and maintain the same weight and a certain fat level that your body needs to be healthy. When you drop below your personal healthy weight/fat range, for example when you diet, your wonderful body/mind will try to pull you back using all kinds of strategies like making you feel hungry, slowing down your metabolism, creating cravings for sweets packed with calories to re-build the fat stores you lose through dieting or restricting what you eat in other ways. How can you tell when you're in your set point zone? It's easy, it's effortless. There is no struggle to maintain it.

Your unique set point is naturally encoded into your body and your mind and you can trust it to do its job without your conscious attention. You know those people who eat what they like, when they want to and never seem to gain or lose an ounce? They are at their happy weight. They often don't know or care how much they weigh. They enjoy food, eat when they are hungry, naturally stop when they are full and hardly ever think about food until they sense they are hungry again. Now and again, they override their body cues and go all out on a big meal with all the trimmings or eat loads of cake in one go but it doesn't phase them. The next day they don't restrict or starve themselves, they just trust their body will tell them when and what to eat next and go with it. Their weight fluctuates now and then and they accept that's normal. Bodies do that when they are in their happy weight range.

TRUSTING YOUR BODY TO RELEASE WEIGHT

As you gain trust in the natural cues of your body you will begin to reconnect and align with your set point coding. When this happens, it can feel unfamiliar or confusing. Women have told me at this stage their experiences included feeling less hungry than usual, instinctively not wanting to eat certain things they found previously hard to resist, not wanting to eat at certain familiar times of the day. Some say they are often eating more than they used to but different foods or food groups that previously they didn't think they liked at all. Others discover they effortlessly prefer fruit to biscuits for a snack, maybe choose a few pieces of dark Swiss chocolate over a couple of Mars bars, or mysteriously find junk food distasteful after years of bingeing on it – and many other shifts that seemed to be happening all by themselves.

When this kind of shift occurs, trust that your gut instinct, your intuition, is overriding your mind's desires and your body is gently aligning you with your goals for a healthy relationship with food and your body. It's a signal that this is a time for it to release weight if that is appropriate for your natural shape and size. Your body knows what you need. It knows your set point and how to get there and stay there. Trust the less hungry days and the other days when you may feel ravenous. Allow yourself to eat what your body, not your

---

Two months into her process, Rachel said:

'Something strange is happening. The other day I didn't feel hungry all morning. I was suspicious. Was I tricking or fooling myself? Was I really not hungry? I decided to trust that my body was telling me I didn't need any food then and my hunger cues would arise eventually. They did after a while and I felt drawn to eat a light lunch and felt surprisingly satisfied after. This is all very new for me but I do feel strangely lighter already without trying so I'm going to keep going with new way of listening to my body and expressing my emotions when I can as it really seems to be working for me'

mind, wants until you're fully satisfied and then stop. Slam the door on your Food Cop, let your body do the talking and it will bring you gently and slowly to the weight that serves and suits you best. Slow release is ideal because your mind and body have time to adjust to the change. Rapid weight release activates starvation signals and panic codes and these prevent weight release automatically, for your survival. Slowly and gently is the way to long term success. Just keep doing what you have been doing: expressing emotions, taking risks, having those conversations, creating strong boundaries, tuning into your hunger and fullness cues, dropping food rules, slamming the door on your Food Cop and you will stay on track.

Now, when you arrive at your personal and unique happy weight, the size and shape you settle at may not tally with the dream vision you created earlier in this process and that is totally fine. That vision was created way back before you practiced all your experiments, became aware of your habits, deleted and installed new codes, and probably learned more about yourself than you imagined you would. That vision may need an upgrade because if you want to live a life free from eating stress and weight obsession, accepting your happy weight is just right for you is a crucial part of the picture. I want to tell you about some interesting discoveries other women have shared after completing this process that may surprise you.

'I FEEL SO MUCH LIGHTER IN MY BEING'

When we end our time together, my clients often say 'I feel like a great weight has lifted from my shoulders. I feel so free. So much lighter in my being'. In fact, it's the most common thing I hear, and it make my heart sing. Through using this process, these wonderful women have dropped a great deal of emotional weight and gained a sense of internal lightness and freedom that can't be measured on a scale, it can only be experienced. Most released physical weight naturally as they boldly released feelings they had previously used food to cover, bury and deny. However, some decided weight loss was not so important after all and that the satisfaction they gained

Franzie called me after twelve weeks of working with me to say: 'Charya it has been amazing. I'm here in my garden feeling content and fat ... this is possible as I've learned that my body fat and my happiness are completely unrelated'.

Tracey emailed me two years after she finished her programme saying,

'I thought I'd let you know that your support was the beginning for me. Since our work together, I've not dieted, I've not weighed myself obsessively, I've not tracked food. I've found a love of exercise for how it makes me feel not for aesthetics and in two years (even during the pandemic and lockdowns) I've had only had a couple of binge eating episodes lasting just a few hours not the days or weeks they used to. Before I would think 'Oh well that's the diet ruined' and would end up in a spiral of shame eating that could go on for days. I just wanted to let you know that because of our work together, when I felt low I have not resorted to self-hatred or trying to eat my way out of feelings. My confidence has soared. I feel fit, happy and great in my skin. I no longer worry about my weight. My work is challenging but I'm going for a promotion and presentations are exciting not daunting any more. That's long-term benefit and I want to say thank you'

from cracking their compulsive eating codes in their minds and relaxing around food and eating was enough.

Critically, these women made radical shifts in areas of their lives that previously they had been trying to deal with through compulsive eating, bingeing, endless dieting, self-shaming and restricting food. And, as they did that their attitude to food, eating and their bodies transformed too. Some left destructive relationships. Some changed jobs, careers, or asked for promotions they had previously avoided. Some allowed their creativity to flourish and dared to exhibit work they have kept hidden for a lifetime in fear of being judged. One sold everything, bought a van and went travelling the world. Some had meaningful, transformational talks with family and loved ones and felt understood, supported and accepted at last. Some finally accepted that their body was absolutely fine and loveable just the way it was and let go of any desire to change it at all.

EXPERIMENT SIXTEEN: UPGRADE YOUR VISION

Review your vision of who you want to be. Is it still in alignment with your current understanding of how you want to feel about yourself, your body, food, eating? Are there any adjustments to make or upgrades to install now you have so much more self-awareness? If so, go ahead and do your magic. However, if like Franzie, you have discovered you are absolutely happy as you are, chuck it in the bin because you don't need a dream if you are already living it!

SELF-ACKNOWLEDMENT

As we are coming to the end of *our* journey together, now is a great time to review and acknowledge all you have achieved so far. You may not have arrived where you want to be yet, but research shows that self-praise works to keep us motivated and on track. Praise boosts self-esteem, criticism diminishes it and self-praise has just the same result.

We compulsive types usually have a perfection code running pretty much all the time. Its critical voice constantly bombards us with putdowns and negative comments however much we have done, tried, changed and shifted. It whispers, 'You should have done better, you haven't tried hard enough, you haven't done it properly, you failed because you didn't do every single experiment, you are useless, you will never crack this, you're not there yet, you're still fat, you haven't lost any or enough weight, you ate a lot of chocolate last night so it's not working, I told you this stupid system was rubbish…' and so it goes on and on. Positively acknowledging what you have achieved – and as often as possible – will close the door on your critical Food Cop and boost your motivation at whatever point you are on your journey.

Every tiny shift forward deserves acknowledgement. Every step counts. Every time you do something, or think something, or say something that cracks a code open a little more is worthy of praise. Now, it's not always easy to lavish praise upon ourselves I know, especially if we have been conditioned to think it's big-headed or were told as kid that only the top marks or the gold cup is good enough. However, you are a kid no longer and you can challenge these unhelpful and downright damaging attitudes. You can consciously choose to make self-praise a new habit, and by now you are an expert on how to build a habit! Just repeat, repeat, repeat. Use the next experiment regularly for an instant self esteem boost!

EXPERIMENT SEVENTEEN:
THE ACKNOWLEDGEMENT GAME

In this experiment only comment on what went well; what you learned, changed and are proud of. Any emotions you released, the time when you didn't eat all the biscuits in the tin because you plucked up the courage to say what you need to say, or you sat with a feeling for a few minutes longer than you ever have before, or you challenged your Food Cop and scraped some food into the bin, or you started walking three times a week, anything at all that marks a shift forward counts. Even if so far, you have managed to read just a few pages of one chapter praise yourself for that. The list of possibilities is endless. Own every success, little or large, and you will build your self-esteem and self-worth every time. To play The Acknowledgment Game, just fill in your answers below.

Three things I changed in my eating behaviour during this process that I am extremely proud of, delighted by, happy about:

1.

2.

3.

Three things I am extremely proud of that I have changed in my non-eating behaviour (e.g., how I speak up for myself now, how I exercise for pleasure now, how I talk to myself now, how I ask for help)

1.

2.

3.

Three small things I have achieved that make me feel a little silly writing about here because they don't seem important enough:
1.

2.

3.

Another three small things I have achieved that make me feel a little silly writing about here because they definitely don't seem important enough:
1.

2.

3.

To make this experiment even more effective, practice it for seven consecutive days with different acknowledgments every time. Or turn it into a 'just before sleeping' habit and drift off to sleep with a mind full of positive thoughts every night.

You can download a Seven-Day Acknowledgement Game via a link in Resources section at the end of this book.

When you are being pestered by your Food Cop the next experiment works wonders.

EXPERIMENT EIGHTEEN: THE MAGIC ARMCHAIR

This experiment takes just three minutes. Read through it first then just go for it. This is how it goes:

1. Make yourself comfortable, set a timer for three minutes and then close your eyes
2. Now imagine you're in an empty room and in front of you there is an open doorway. The space behind the doorway is completely dark
3. Now imagine an armchair on one side of the room. You can choose which side it is on and you can make it any kind of armchair you like: any colour, any fabric
4. Now before long a thought is going to pop into your mind
5. Imagine this thought comes from the darkness and in through the doorway and without judging it as positive or negative, or what it relates to, simply greet the thought and lead it over to the armchair and place it on the chair
6. Now, bring your attention back to the doorway and wait for the next thought to arise and repeat the action again. Greet the thought and gently lead it over to the armchair and then look back at the doorway again
7. Repeat this process for the next three minutes

Practice this experiment twice daily and you will discover it can work wonders.

MOVE IT, MOVE IT, MOVE IT!

Bodies are designed to move and exercise. Create a moving habit. Not because you think it will help you lose weight or tone up but simply because it feels good. Try out different kinds of movement – gentle exercise like walking or swimming is great for the body and the mind. If your movement is limited or you would love to go swimming but a pool isn't available close by or within your budget, search out gentle stretching exercises, chair yoga or Pilates on YouTube. Or my favourite after walking – dancing! I just put on some music and go for it. Dancing brings joy to the body and soul within moments of prancing around plus it can work up a sweat and costs nothing. What's not to love? If you prefer something more intense, there is always the gym, or weights and stretch band routines on YouTube and countless other systems, classes, sports clubs everywhere. However, the most important thing to remember is that you focus on enjoying moving your body. Drop the 'no pain, no gain' idea. If you choose something that gives you pleasure, you are much more likely to keep doing it.

GRATITUDE

Gratitude, like self-acknowledgement, is a powerful ally in silencing the critical Food Cop and any other unhelpful critical voices that may hang around in your head. The next experiment is designed to engender an attitude of gratitude to your body – however far you have come along your journey.

EXPERIMENT NINETEEN: GRATITUDE

You will need a full-length mirror or at least one that is long enough to see most of your body, a few minutes of undisturbed time and a little courage. You can stand or sit.

1. With your eyes open, stand or sit in front of your mirror and just let your gaze **slowly** run over your body from head to toe and then back up again
2. Notice what you are feeling and thinking. Notice your criticisms, what you like and what you don't like, what you want to avoid or skim over
3. Now close your eyes for a moment or two and take a few deep breaths
4. Open your eyes again. Look at your reflection and begin to thank your body for all it does for you every day. Thank it for breathing, for your heart beating, for the blood that pulses round and into every tiny bit of you every nanosecond. Thank all your organs, glands, muscles, tendons, bones, nerves, skin, hair and nails. Thank everything. Thank your incredible mind that keeps on working to protect you and to keep your body going however much you send it messages of despair and hopelessness and maybe even self-hatred now and then
5. Finally, take another deep breath and relax

This can be a very challenging exercise but it can be profoundly moving and transformational when it is repeated regularly. You will discover you can gradually learn to love yourself just the way you are now and however much you change going forward. You are enough. You have always been enough and you will always be enough regardless of your shape, size, weight now and in your future.

Your next and final experiment can transform your experience of your day, every day.

EXPERIMENT TWENTY: FIRST THING EVERY MORNING

Each morning, as you wake up, lie in your bed for a few moments and practice this short meditation.

1. Close your eyes again, relax, take one deep breath and exhale fully
2. Now, on the next breath inhale for four counts, hold that breath for seven counts, then exhale for eight counts making an 'ah' sound as you let the breath go
3. Repeat this for three rounds more and then keeping your eyes closed, imagine or sense your body just the way it is as you continue to breathe easily and comfortably
4. Now still with your eyes closed, take your awareness all the way down to the tip of your toes and then let it slowly, gently float up all the way through your body to the top of your head
5. Say to yourself 'I am contented with my body. I love and accept my body just the way it is' and repeat this mantra to yourself three times
6. Then when you're ready, get up and go about whatever it is you will be doing, keeping your new mantra in your mind
7. When you notice you've forgotten to keep your mantra in your mind, just repeat it, with no judgement, and continue with your day

It doesn't matter how many times you remember or forget. This experiment is not a test, it's just an awareness exercise. Even if you don't believe the statement practice it anyway. See how you feel and what happens over time as you repeat and reprogramme your mind to love yourself day after day.

CHAPTER 8 KEY POINTS

- To get to a place where we feel happy in our skin and our lives are not ruled by food, we must understand that it's not about the food at all. It's about so much more

- People come in all shapes and sizes and your natural, or 'set point', is an individual, balanced, harmonised state that is biologically and uniquely right for you

- As you gain trust in the natural cues of your body you will begin to reconnect and align with your set point coding

- After completing this process, some people decided weight loss is not so important after all and that the satisfaction they gained from cracking their compulsive eating codes in their minds and relaxing around food and eating is enough

- Praise boosts self-esteem, criticism diminishes it and self-praise has just the same result. Always!

CRACK YOUR CODE

1. Practice Experiment Sixteen: Upgrade Your Vision. Review your 'Dream You' and uplevel it as often as you choose – or if you are like Franzie and you have discovered you are absolutely happy as you are, chuck it in the bin because you are already living your dream

2. Practice Experiment Seventeen: The Acknowledgement Game for seven consecutive days and go on to make it a before sleeping habit. Drift off to sleep every night with a mind full of positive thoughts

3. Practice Experiment Eighteen: The Magic Armchair. Practice it twice daily and discover how it can work wonders

4. Practice Experiment Nineteen: Gratitude. Practice gratitude regularly for gratitude is your most powerful ally in silencing your Food Cop

5. Practice Experiment Twenty: First Thing Every Morning.
    As you wake, lie in bed for a few precious minutes and
    appreciate your body. Practice your mantra and keep it in
    your mind. And remember – when you forget to remember
    that's fine. Just remember it again and repeat it
6. Continue to journal and listen to your self-hypnosis
    recording as often as you choose. Transformation is an on-
    going process
7. Always, always, always treat yourself with loving kindness and
    honour your body every day

9

MOVING FORWARD

My top tips

1. Stay active: This process is based on the scientific model which means actively trying the experiments – testing the ideas, not just reading about them or theorising – is the *only* way to find out if they are valid and can bring you the results you want. So, if you haven't fully engaged so far, go back when you are ready and do what you didn't do or try what you didn't try. In no particular order, just follow your intuition. If you are aware that you avoided certain chapters or experiments, be curious and choose to return and look into what you've been avoiding. Often there are pearls of wisdom waiting to reveal themselves in those glossed-over pages

2. Invest in yourself: Always buy the best you can afford (another one of my mother's sayings and it's a great one) whether that be clothes, books, nourishing food, therapy or whatever else floats your boat. If you think you don't deserve to, or that it's a waste of money, just remember how much you have spent on diets that didn't work, diet club memberships, diet foods you hated, meal replacement drinks, diet pills, exercise regimes, fitness paraphernalia and gym passes you never used or completed, never mind all the money you may have spent on food for binges

3. Wear what you love: Wear what fits. What feels great. Don't wait until you lose weight or until you think you deserve to wear beautiful clothes. Don't wait to be thin to wear that slinky dress, wide belt, shorts, bikini, skinny jeans or whatever else your inner Fashion Cop says you shouldn't. Your body is always bikini ready! Don't keep clothes in your

wardrobe that you know you will never get into unless you starve yourself. Take them to a charity shop and stock up on new stuff that looks good on you while you are there if you are financially able to

4. Eat like the French: Get emotional about eating. Chuck out the food rules. Eat slowly. Enjoy every morsel. Relish it, love it and let it go. Trust your natural hunger cues to tell you when it's time to eat again

5. Boundaries: Be bold. Create clear boundaries and remember: people treat us like we treat ourselves so treat yourself with respect and you will receive it

6. Vision: Keep your focus on what you want – not what you don't want. Stay in alignment with your dream. Say yes to anything that takes you closer to embodying and being her and no to everything that isn't in alignment with that

7. Joy: Be clear about what makes you genuinely happy, what brings you joy. What's genuinely important and valuable to you in your life? Express it, do it, live it, love it

8. Kindness: Be patient, gentle and compassionate with yourself. Speak with loving kindness to yourself always

9. Spread Kindness: Spread kindness and compassion to others

10. Please Remember: You are enough. You have always been enough. You will always be enough – always and forever

MY 'WHY'

The sense of freedom that comes when we stop hating our bodies and dare to trust our natural intuition is priceless. To me, as a life-long feminist, loving ourselves in a world that feeds on our insecurities is a truly revolutionary act. The ultimate rebellion in a culture that tells us we are not, and never will be, *enough* the way we are.

This was my 'why', my reason for writing this book. My dream, my big vision, is that every woman everywhere who struggles with eating and body issues can refresh the sense of freedom around food and liberation about their bodies that is their birthright. And, as I can't possibly personally reach all the millions of women who suffer – often in silence – I am creating a vision that this book can. Hopefully it will help many, many women to feel less alone and hopeless. I hope it has helped you.

With deep gratitude, please remember always:

You are enough.
You have always been enough.
You will always be enough.

Charya

Resources

The links to your resources:

Experiment 1: **The Seven Day Eating Log** (chapter 4, page 31), and Experiment 17: **The Acknowledgement Game** (chapter 8, page 98) can both be downloaded from:

www.charyahilton.com/resources   or scan:

Your hypnosis recording: The Quantum Jump (chapter 3, page 26)
www.charyahilton.com/crack-your-code   or scan:

Waiver

Do not listen to this recording while driving or operating machinery. By listening to this hypnosis recording you hereby release Charya Hilton from any liability or claims that could be made against her concerning your mental and/or physical well-being.

You understand that I, Charya Hilton, am not a licensed medical practitioner, physician or psychologist of any kind and that this hypnosis recording should not be considered a replacement for the advice and/or services of a psychiatrist, psychotherapist or doctor. If you are under the care of a medical practitioner and/or on any medication do not make any adjustments without the approval of your doctor. If in any doubt, please contact your physician.

ABOUT THE AUTHOR

Charya Hilton is an internationally accredited Master Coach, Hypnotherapist and Integrative Nutritional Health Coach.

For over twenty-five years she has been helping women – and men – successfully overcome chronic dieting, binge eating, compulsive and emotional eating and go on to maintain a healthy relationship with food and their bodies free from food stress and body shame.

Her personal journey to food freedom began when she was in her early twenties. Severely anorexic then subsequently suffering from secretive compulsive eating and bulimia for years, she was almost at breaking point when she discovered a group being run by Susie Orbach (of *Fat is a Feminist Issue* fame) and plucked up the courage to go along. It was her first breakthrough. She began to understand through the therapeutic work in that group that she could be free from the despair she was enduring if she was prepared to dedicate herself to finding out all she could about the root causes of her eating problems, who she really was underneath all that pain – and who she could be. She went on a personal journey of self-discovery, daring to let go of dieting and binging, and over time learned to trust the natural wisdom of her body. As she did that her body eventually came to rest at her unique, natural, healthy size and shape.

Charya realised she wanted to help other people to be free from fighting with food and their bodies too. She trained in various kinds of personal growth work, and individual and group therapy graduating as a Professional Performance Coach, Neuro-Linguistic Programming Practitioner, Hypnotherapist, Master Coach, and Integrative Nutrition Health Coach.

She runs courses, workshops and seminars in Food Freedom, Confidence and Manifesting and has a successful coaching practice as a Master Confidence Coach and Hypnotherapist. She lives in Newquay, Cornwall UK.

You can find her online at **www.charyahilton.com**

Reviews

I love this book so much. Charya is not only a fabulous person, she is an amazing professional and true expert on this topic. I am honoured to be a colleague and friend. Like me, she understands the food and body struggle from first-hand experience. She understands the toll it takes on your body, mind, and soul. But she also knows what it takes to be FREE and she can help you find your freedom too! If you are sick and tired of the exhausting cycle of overeating and then fearfully restricting food, this book is meant for you. Charya does a beautiful job explaining how we end up in a compulsive relationship with food in the first place, and then page by page she holds your hand through a transformational process that can bring you to your freedom if you choose to take her hand. This book will change your life if you are ready to embrace it and apply it!

Rebecca Laurel-Hill. Registered Dietitian-Nutritionist

This book is brilliantly written. I really adore the practical exercises throughout the book because ultimately implementation is what is going to help people break out of the vicious cycles of yo-yo dieting and compulsive, emotional and binge eating rather than intellectual knowledge. And the exercises are varied enough that even if for some reason someone doesn't resonate with one, they will definitely resonate with another. There is an exercise for every taste and every need.

Ines Padar. Aka The Imposter Syndrome Terminator

The structure of this book really works. It is clearly laid out and logical to follow, whilst still completely having Charya's voice and open clear style. At the end of each chapter there is a little work to do which means the book cannot, and should not, be swallowed up in one sitting. I did wonder how Charya might be able to convey her magic and the wholeness of her approach in a book but I think she has really nailed it!

Sasha Avoscan. Successful Code Cracker

This is an amazing book. I really like how Charya uses the code cracking theme all the way through. An excellent, easy flowing read which is somehow challenging yet supportive. I am sure it will help many people out there.

Alice Maggs. Health Educationalist

Printed in Great Britain
by Amazon

32638951R00069